Yáng Jìzhōu's 楊繼州

針 灸 大 成

The Great Compendium of Acupuncture and Moxibustion

Zhēn Jiǔ Dà Chéng

Volume I

Sabine Wilms, Ph.D.

The Chinese Medicine Database
www.cm-db.com
Portland, Oregon

The Great Compendium of Acupuncture and Moxibustion

針灸大成

Zhēn Jiǔ Dà Chéng

Volume I

Sabine Wilms

Copyright © 2010 The Chinese Medicine Database

1017 SW Morrison #306
Portland, OR 97205 USA

COMP designation original Chinese work and English translation

Cover Design by Jonathan Schell L.Ac.
Artwork courtesy of the Needham Research Institute
Library of Congress Cataloging-in-Publication Data:

Yang, Jizhou, fl.
  [The Great Compendium of Acupuncture and Moxibustion. English]
  Zhen Jiu Da Cheng = The Great Compendium of Acupuncture and
  Moxibustion/ translation Sabine Wilms
    p. cm.
  Includes Index.
  ISBN 978-0-9799552-2-8 (alk. paper)
  Medicine, Chinese   I. Wilms, Sabine. II. Title: The
  Great Compendium of Acupuncture and Moxibustion.
  III. Title: Vol. I

International Standard Book Number (ISBN): 978-0-9799552-2-8
Printed in the United States of America

Contents

Translation

Volume I

Contents

Contents

Contents

Contents

Illustrations

Indices

針
灸
大
成
・
卷
之
一

The *Zhēn Jiǔ Dà Chéng*, a Brief History of Acupuncture and Moxibustion, and the Importance of the Classics
by Sabine Wilms

Why do we read, translate, and publish the historical classics of Chinese medicine? Why are some of us in the field of Chinese medicine (including practitioners, translators, patients, and publishers) convinced that a text composed more than 400 years ago will positively contribute to actual clinical practice in our contemporary world? Why should you as a well-rounded, educated practitioner of Chinese medicine in our busy modern world care about the experiences and opinions of a physician so distant in space and time? What could the ancient sages possibly have to teach us? Answering these questions is not an easy task, but that fact should not deter us from engaging in this important conversation. These questions are even more pressing in the case of this first volume of the *Great Compendium of Acupuncture and Moxibustion*,[1] consisting as it does primarily of quotations from texts that were yet another 1500 years, give or take, removed from the compilation date of the *Great Compendium* in 1601. If we draw a parallel to the history of biomedical science, how many medical schools do you know that require future heart surgeons or oncologists to read the Greek Hippocratic Corpus (compiled several centuries before the Common Era), Galen's writings on anatomy (second century CE, translated into Latin and popularized in medieval Europe by the Belgian physician Andreas Vesalius in the sixteenth century), or the *Canon of Medicine* by the Persian physician and philosopher Avicenna (Ibn Sīnā) from the tenth century, which combined his extensive personal experience with his deep knowledge of Islamic, Greek, Indian, and Mesopotamic medicine and was used as a core textbook in many medieval universities?

Regardless of whether we practice in what we often simplistically refer to as the "Chinese" or the "Western" paradigm of medicine, consciously and intentionally or not, most of us are steeped in an approach to science and medicine that is rooted in our Greco-Roman heritage and firmly believes in the unstoppable progress and development of medical knowledge. The history of modern medicine is marked by a more and more sophisticated understanding of the workings of the human body and increasingly effective treatment options. Usually, this progress is related to and made possible by theoretical discoveries (by the likes of Darwin, Einstein, and other "heroic" thinkers) and technological inventions (penicillin, x-rays, MRIs...) that make it superfluous to look back at the "primitive" practices of our ancestors who lacked access to these insights or tools. And it is important here to note that this attitude informs not only contemporary "Western" medicine, more

---

1. In the following, abbreviated as "Great Compendium."

accurately perhaps referred to as "cosmopolitan" or "bio-" medicine, but also the version of contemporary Chinese medicine that is known in English as "Traditional Chinese Medicine" (TCM), namely the medicine that has been created and promoted by the People's Republic of China since roughly the 1950s, which is the direct or indirect source of most publications and research on Chinese medicine in Western languages.

Without giving a full-blown account of the differences between Chinese and European models of scientific progress and the production of knowledge, which would far transcend the framework of this short introduction, it is essential that we understand the very different role played by the classics in the context of traditional Chinese science.[2] To fully appreciate the significance of the classics in all aspects of Chinese thought, and hence also in an acupuncture text like the *Great Compendium*, we must turn our gaze all the way back to early Confucian philosophy. As one possible response to the social and political upheavals before the formation of a unified Chinese empire under the Qín and Hàn dynasties in the third century BCE, Confucius and his followers formulated a sentiment that has continued to remain salient throughout China's long history, namely the idealization of a golden age of sagely insight and harmony in the long distant past. In the age before youtube and digital recordings, the wisdom of this ancient past could best be accessed in the less enlightened presence by means of the early writings known as "classics" (*jīng* 經), as abstruse as they might be. As a result, the knowledge of the past expressed in the classics has always enjoyed a revered status in China that is quite the opposite of our own attitude—in the scientific context—of benign condescension toward the great writings from the Greco-Roman, Arabic, or medieval pre-Enlightenment periods.

Of course, to read this old text as a source of clinically valuable information requires a very different set of attitudes toward medical practice and the self-identity of the physician or "healer." It is certainly the case that you can now obtain a degree of Chinese medicine in a few years, call yourself a "licensed acupuncturist" (L.Ac.) or "Doctor of Oriental Medicine" (D.O.M.), and establish a thriving clinical practice by mastering the basics of such technical skills as simple pulse diagnosis and needling, and memorizing channel and point locations, major patterns and diseases, and a limited amount of information on individual herbs and well-known formulas. You will be able to contribute to your patients' well-being by providing a low-cost effective alternative to biomedical care, whose prohibitive costs and sometimes formidable side-effects make it less and less desirable for many people, especially in the US. Nevertheless, as this book will hopefully begin to show you, Chinese medicine can and should be so much more than the technical skill of matching diseases to treatment plans in a paint-by-number style. To quote the eleventh-century text *Effective Prescriptions of Sū and Shěn* (*Sū Shěn liáng fāng* 蘇沈良方), "Treating a disease has five difficulties: differentiating the disease, treating the disease, drinking the medicinals, compounding the formula, and distinguishing between the medicinals [in the formula]."[3]

---

2. For a more detailed account, see Geoffrey Lloyd and Nathan Sivin, *The Way and the Word: Science and Medicine in Early China and Greece* (Yale University Press, 2002).

3. I am indebted to Yaron Seidman for bringing this evocative quote to my attention. The transla-

針
灸
大
成
・
卷
之
一

Sūn Sīmiǎo and the Ideal of the Great Physician

Looked at from a different angle, the often-cited chapter by Sūn Sīmiǎo on "The Professional Practice of the Great Physician" outlines the basic requirements in the training of a "great physician."[4] The first item on Sūn's shopping list of medical training consists of familiarity with the major medical classics: theoretical treatises, books on acupuncture, moxibustion, and pulse diagnosis, and materia medica and formularies. The next major item on his list, though, might surprise you: You must master the various techniques of divination in order to predict people's fate (such as calendrical techniques, astrology, physiognomy, plastromancy (i.e. turtle shell divination), the *Classic of Changes* (*Yì jīng* 易經) etc., to avoid being "like a traveler at night without eyesight, blindly stumbling to your death." Next you must study the prescriptions contained in Sūn's book, the *Essential Prescriptions Worth a Thousand in Gold for Every Emergency* (*Bèi jí qiān jīn yào fāng* 備急千金要方), by "fixing your mind on them, pinching them tightly as if with tweezers and grinding them down like ink stones." As if this program weren't enough for one lifetime, you must "wade and hunt through the general literature," explained as the Confucian classics, the Dynastic Histories, the Buddhist sutras, and the Daoist philosophers, to cultivate humaneness and righteousness; understand the ways of the past and present; foster the virtues of compassion, sympathy, joy and abandonment; and physically transform your body by means of longevity practices, respectively. When, lastly, you have investigated the astrological details of the planets and stars, celestial patterns, and cosmological changes in the framework of correlative thinking, "there will be no obstacles in your way of medicine, and it will be characterized by perfection of both skill and beauty."

After having completed this program, you must follow certain ethical requirements in your daily practice, such as an attitude of self-possession and concentration, a dignified appearance, equal treatment of all patients with no regard to wealth, gender, status, nature of ailment, or potential rewards, and a life of utmost devotion to easing the suffering of your fellow humans regardless of physical discomforts, while abstaining from luxuries and from criticizing your fellow physicians. Further down in the same volume, in the chapter on the "Absolute Sincerity of the Great Physician," Sūn Sīmiǎo states that "the fools of the world study formulas for three years and yet we can say that there is not a disease under heaven that they are able to treat. After treating disease for three years, they finally become aware that no formula under heaven exists that they are able to use. For

---

tion is my own.

4. From Sūn Sīmiǎo, *Bèi Jí Qiān Jīn Yào Fāng*, vol. 1. Translated and explained in Wilms, *Bèi Jí Qiān Jīn Yào Fāng*, pp. 13-14. Here you will also find a discussion of Sūn Sīmiǎo's biography and life work to contextualize the information given here further.

this reason, students must absolutely acquaint themselves to the greatest extent with the origins of medicine, studying tirelessly with absolute diligence. They may not recklessly repeat rumors and then claim that this is all there is to the Way of Medicine! Deep indeed is their self-delusion!"[5]

The reason for my citing the famous Sūn Sīmiǎo here in such detail is that he has so masterfully outlined the ideals that a practitioner of Chinese medicine should aspire to; ideals that, I believe, can still serve us well as guideposts in today's medicine. As much as we celebrate Sūn Sīmiǎo these days, the true extent of his ideals tends to be woefully overlooked by contemporary practitioners, students, and educators in their rush to provide a satisfactory and sorely needed alternative and complement to biomedical care. As a result, the full potential of Chinese medicine, the ART behind the CRAFT, the true essence of this ancient treasure-trove of knowledge on the human body and its interactions with the natural, social, and macrocosmic environments in the ever-changing transformations of qì, often remains unexplored and neglected. As we can see from the quotes above, Sūn Sīmiǎo already warned of the detrimental effects of intellectual laziness, ignorance, lack of moral standards, and greed on medical practice. How much more difficult it is today when 99.99% of Chinese medical texts are only available to those of us fortunate enough be able to read and understand classical Chinese medical literature! Throughout the history of Chinese medicine, medical practitioners and authors have bemoaned the chronic shortage of true sages and "great physicians" in the flesh, at whose feet we could learn by example. As a response, they have always turned to the ancient writings and have compiled and composed medical literature based on their understanding of the classics, ideally through the filter of their personal experiences. And this is precisely the way in which Yáng Jìzhōu created the *Great Compendium*.

The Origins of Acupuncture
Early Manuscripts

To contextualize the *Great Compendium* further, let us take a very cursory look at the roots and development of acupuncture (and to a lesser extent, moxibustion) up to the point in time, when Yáng Jìzhōu composed his grand opus. Given how far removed the origins of these therapeutic practices are from our own time and culture, it should come as no surprise that they are still shrouded in much mystery and controversy. The dating obviously depends on how narrowly we define the practices and theories behind them and how willing we are to treat mythologic records as historical facts. For the purposes of our discussion here, I define acupuncture rather narrowly as the insertion of needles at specific points on the patient's body for the purpose of manipulating the flow of qì in the vessels. Given this definition, contrary to the unsubstantiated claims found so often in both Chinese and international textbooks, archaeological discoveries of manuscripts and

---

5. Ibid. vol. 1.

tools in conjunction with received texts suggest that we situate the origins of acupuncture not in the distant mythological past more than five thousand years ago or even the Neolithic period,[6] but more realistically around the beginning of the Common Era. To be sure, we have earlier written and material evidence for sharp objects being inserted into the body in China in a medical context, most notably in the famous so-called Mǎwángduī manuscripts, found in a tomb in Southern China that was closed in 168 BCE. Nevertheless, the insertion of needles into the body is here used not in the context of manipulating the flow of qì in the vessels but of opening purulent ulcers and abscesses. Since the therapeutic application of sharp objects for the purpose of lancing abscesses or letting blood is also common in many other cultures, I do not consider it acupuncture in the strictest (and contemporary) sense of the word.

It appears that Chinese healers first stabbed and beat patients with objects like lancing stones or peach wood arrows to exorcise demons. As unwelcome guests who had taken up residence in the human body and were held responsible for all sorts of conditions, they had to be intimidated, verbally threatened, and, if necessary, literally beaten or stabbed to persuade the malignant spirits to leave the body of their suffering host. Given the religious significance of wormwood (artemisia, also called mugwort or moxa, from the Japanese pronunciation), it is likely that the practice of moxibustion (lit. the burning of moxa) had its origin in the same notions of demonic medicine. Leaving a detailed discussion to more specialized medical historians, for the purpose of this book it is important to note that pre-Hàn medical texts contain instructions for exorcising demons by stabbing and beating them as well as for lancing abscesses and ulcers with sharpened objects, namely *biān* 砭 ("lancing stones") and *zhēn* 針 ("needles").

A separate textual genre, which Elisabeth Hsu calls "Cauterization Classics" (*jiǔ jīng* 灸經) and of which two examples are included in the Mǎwángduī medical corpus, discusses eleven vessels, associated with gradations of yīn and yáng, in terms of their visually perceived courses and associated pathologies, to be treated simply by means of "cauterization," i.e. moxibustion. It is important to note that we do not yet find any traces of the notion of a continuous circulation of qì through a network of interconnected vessels, or even an association of the vessels with a movement of qì contained therein at all! Nor do we find in these treatises on vessels and vessel pathology any reference to points or holes nor to needles and acupuncture as a means of treating them![7]

In yet another group of writings that Vivienne Lo convincingly associates with the tradition of

---

6. See for example http://en.wikipedia.org/wiki/Acupuncture. The same entry also dates the composition of the *Inner Classic of the Yellow Emperor* (*Huáng Dì Nèi Jīng*) to 305-204 BCE, which is most certainly several centuries too early.

7. For a complete translation of the medical manuscripts discovered at Mǎwángduī, see Donald Harper, *Early Chinese Medical Literature: The Mawangdui Medical Manuscripts* (Kegan Paul International, 2000). For more information on the notions of the vessels and qì in early Chinese medicine, see Elisabeth Hsu's and Vivienne Lo's contributions to the section on "Mài" and "qì" in the Western Hàn in Hsu, ed., *Innovation in Chinese Medicine* (Cambridge University Press, 2001).

"nurturing life" (*yǎng shēng* 養生), lastly, we find a discourse on increasing or "extending" qì, primarily by means of sexual and breath cultivation in a subjectively experienced and poetically described body. The rich language we find here to describe bodily locations and sensations, related to the personal subjective experience of qì as a response to sexual or breath-related stimulation, was, according to Lo, adopted in the later medical classics in the naming of acumoxa point locations; in other words, the acumoxa literature that we find in the classics several centuries later originated in the conflation of two separate literary genres, one on nurturing life and the other on vessel pathology, which predate the beginning of the Common Era by ca. 2-3 centuries.

The Transmitted Classics

As tempting as it may be, we have to skip here over the material discoveries of archaeology and references to needling and vessels in the biography of the physician Biǎn Què 扁鵲 in the *Records of a Historian* (*Shǐ jì* 史記) from the first century CE.[8] After extensively researching the various textual layers of the *Inner Classic of the Yellow Emperor*, Paul Unschuld has convincingly argued that while some might have been composed as early as the second or even third century BCE, the text was most likely compiled into something roughly resembling its present form no earlier than the first to second century CE. Even more significant, the most authentic edition transmitted to us today is the one that Wáng Bīng 王冰 presented to the Táng emperor in 762. Most likely, Wáng Bīng in fact added as much as a full third, namely chapters 66-71 and 74, which are the chapters that describe the doctrine of *wǔ yùn liù qì* 五運六氣 ("five movements and six qì"). Be that as it may, Volker Scheid has argued from his perspective of classical medicine that "by 280 A.D., all of the foundational texts of the tradition had been written."[9] While this statement, in my opinion, overlooks the key role of clinically applied literature, most notably formulary texts, it is certainly true that the major theoretical notions in classical Chinese medicine such as qì, yīn-yáng, the system of the five viscera and six bowels, the channels and network vessels (*jīng luò* 經絡), pulse diagnosis, and correlative thinking on the basis of macrocosm-microcosm correspondences, had been formulated by then. And the two key texts in this development are without doubt the above-mentioned *Inner Classic of the Yellow Emperor* (*Huáng dì nèi jīng* 黃帝內經), consisting of two parts: *Plain Questions* (*Sù wèn* 素問) and *Divine Pivot* (*Líng shū* 靈樞), and the *Classic of Difficult Issues* (*Nàn jīng* 難經), which are precisely the texts that provide the majority of material for this first volume of the *Great Compendium*.

To put it very simplistically, the *Inner Classic of the Yellow Emperor* introduces,—and the *Classic of*

---

8. For an excellent discussion of the notions of *mài* and *qì* in the *Records of the Historian* (*Shǐ Jì*), see Elisabeth Hsu's article on "Pulse Diagnostics in the Western Han: how *mài* and *qì* determine *bìng*," in Hsu, *Innovation in Chinese Medicine*, pp. 51-91.

9. Volker Scheid, *Currents of Tradition in Chinese Medicine 1626-2006* (Eastland Press, 2007), p. 35.

針灸大成・卷之一

Difficult Issues refines,—a theoretical understanding of the human body as a microcosm that is constantly transforming in response to the changes of qì occurring in the macrocosm of its natural and social environment. The texts were intended as guides to medically inclined readers from among the literate scholar-bureaucrat elite of early Chinese society on how to "nurture life," i.e., to cultivate the body so as to maintain or restore the natural harmony between yīn and yáng and between the microcosm of the body and the macrocosm at large. They certainly also lay out the key rules of clinical practice that Chinese medicine is still based on, in terms of diagnosis (pulse taking, observation of the patient's complexion, posture, movements, behavior, etc., smelling, questioning the patient, etc.), pathology (interior versus exterior, construction versus defense, invasion of external pathogens and internal imbalances, progression of disease through the viscera and bowels, etc.), and therapy (acupuncture, moxibustion, medicinal preparations, diet, exercises, etc.).

But at the root of both texts, we can find the ideal of "treating disease before it arises" (*zhì wéi bìng* 治未病) and the hope to teach a system of medicine that worked primarily by prevention, early recognition, and gentle adjustment, before diseases had entered the body deeply enough to necessitate drastic interventions. The main tool for interpreting past changes in the patient's history, recognizing current interactions with and influences from the macrocosmic environment, and predicting future developments was the doctrine of the five phases (*wǔ xíng* 五行: wood, fire, earth, metal, water). The balance of the five phases and yīn and yáng allowed the human body to maintain its smoothly flowing equilibrium as a complex interrelated and interdependent network of storage and administrative centers (i.e., the viscera and bowels) with transportation pathways (the channels and network vessels) for the intake, transport, and elimination of vital substances and information (qì, blood, and essence, construction and defense qì, and the nutrients derived from liquids and solids in the diet).

Significant for the development of acupuncture theory specifically, these texts established a theory of qì as continuously circulating through the channels and their paired viscera and bowels in a predictable progression, speed, and direction. The movement of this pulse (*mài* 脈) could be read by means of pulse-taking at the three wrist positions (*cùn* 寸, *guān* 關, and *chǐ* 尺) that are still used today. To complete this theory of medicine, acupuncture and moxibustion became the therapeutic means of choice for manipulating this flow by resolving blockages, stimulating flow, draining excess, and supplementing insufficiencies. While not integrated in any systematic fashion, many of the 365 points claimed to exist in the theory are mentioned by name and sometimes described in terms of vague locations or indications.

The next and final step in the development of classical acupuncture theory followed soon afterwards in the form of the *A to Z Classic of Acupuncture and Moxibustion* (*Zhēn jiǔ jiǎ yǐ jīng* 針灸甲乙經), composed around 259 by Huángfǔ Mì 皇甫謐. The first text to be devoted exclusively to acupuncture and moxibustion, it mentions 349 points in a systematic list, in each case giving their location, indications, and preferred needling techniques. Also included in the book are treatment instructions and point selections for 150 diseases and lists of contraindicated points and synonyms for point names. And it is probably indeed fair to say, at least in the context of acupuncture and moxibustion, that the composition of this text does in fact mark the end of the highly creative period during which the theoretical foundations were laid.

Subsequent Developments

This fact should never lead us to ignore the following centuries, especially of course the famous Sūn Sīmiǎo and his grand work in the seventh century, which also has much to say about acupuncture and moxibustion. It is simply that they are not directly pertinent to the topic at hand and we can therefore, in the context of this short introduction, jump ahead several centuries to the year 1026 in the Sòng period. This year marks another significant stage in the development of acupuncture: As part of the standardization and specialization that took place in many fields of medicine as the result of large-scale publication and education projects officially sponsored by the court, a life-sized figure was created out of bronze under the auspices of imperial medical bureau. This figure was covered with tiny holes in the location of the standard acumoxa points and was accompanied by an explanatory manual that identified the points by name and listed their indications. The purpose of this figure was to train and examine medical students by having them needle the statue after it was prepared by being coated with wax and filled with water. When students inserted a needle in the correct location, the needle went through the predrilled holes in the bronze and water spurted out. When they tried inserting needles in locations that were not officially designated acumoxa points, they simply bent the needle, unable to penetrate the bronze. Just for the purpose of comparison, this statue and the accompanying manual only recorded 354 points, that is, exactly 5 points more than the *A to Z Classic of Acupuncture and Moxibustion* from the third century CE.[10]

There are two reasons why the creation of this statue and accompanying textbook is significant: First, the quite extensive devotion of resources involved shows the important role accorded by the imperial court to the practice of acupuncture and moxibustion, and to the proper education therein. Clearly, the Chinese government was highly invested in promoting the skill of correctly identifying a set number of standardized points, all for the benefit of improving the health of the population at large. And just as clearly, it was aware of the danger of acupuncture and moxibustion being employed by insufficiently trained practitioners unable to identify the full number of points correctly. The second noteworthy fact here is the mere existence of this level of consensus on the specific identity of acumoxa points and the small amount of change that took place between the third and the eleventh century in China. Based on this consensus, the bronze statue was invented as an ingenious method for testing a practitioner's ability to properly localize acumoxa points, an issue that has vexed CM practitioners, educators, and researchers up to the present, as evidenced for ex-

---

10. I thank Iven Tao for sharing this observation in his unpublished manuscript, *Physiology of Acupuncture: Anatomy of a Historical Construct.*

ample by the current discussion on applying the scientific methodology of randomized controlled studies in acupuncture research trials, which involve the questionable use of "sham" acupuncture and the insertion of needles at "non-acupuncture" points.

The *Great Compendium of Acupuncture and Moxibustion*

As we can see from this brief example, the history of acupuncture after the foundational period is thus not marked by grand path-breaking discoveries that revolutionized previously existing practices and theories, but rather by increasing sophistication, standardization, and refinement in both theory and clinical application. If that is the case, what is it that makes the *Great Compendium* such an important text? Why is it that this text was chosen by seventeenth-century European Jesuit missionaries, merchants, and later also physicians as their key source to be translated into Latin and thereby sparked a wave of interest in Chinese medicine and the practice of acupuncture all over Europe that was based on the understanding of Chinese medicine as represented in this text? As late as the early twentieth century, what is even now considered one of the key texts on Chinese acupuncture in a Western language, the enormous *L'Acuponcture Chinoise* composed by the Frenchman George Soulie de Morant after his return from China to France in 1917, still gives credit to the *Great Compendium* as one of its key sources! To better understand the continuing significance of this text, let us look at the circumstances of its composition, the background of the author, and briefly review its content.

Published in 1601 by a true scholar-physician named Yáng Jìzhōu, the *Great Compendium* was composed at a time of wide-spread political turmoil during the declining years of the Míng dynasty, shortly before its take-over by the Manchus and the founding of the Qīng dynasty in 1636. For the larger context in the history of medicine, let me quote Paul Unschuld: "The diversity of schools and their conflicting views during the Míng and Qīng [sic.] periods convey the impression that the conceptual framework of systematic correspondence at this time was nothing more than a complex labyrinth, in which those thinkers seeking solutions to medical questions wandered aimlessly in all directions, lacking any orientation, and unable to find a feasible way out."[11] Once again, this was a period during which many intellectuals blamed the doctrines popular in the more recent past, during this time most notably Sòng Neoconfucianism, for the chaos and suffering they witnessed in their own lifetime. As an alternative, they advocated a return to the ideals of the classical Hàn and Táng civilizations. Many intellectuals, including medical thinkers, turned their backs to the empty philosophizing that had become so popular in Neoconfucianism and instead devoted themselves to an individual search for wisdom in the writings of the ancient past, for a new and "true" understanding of the classics, aided by their personal experiences and the direct observation of the

---

11. Paul U. Unschuld, *History of Ideas* (University of California Press, 1985), p. 197

external reality in their human, natural, and macrocosmic environment.

In medicine, Yáng Jìzhōu's life story nicely illustrates this tendency to return to the classics, but with an understanding of the human body that was also enriched by the author's clinical experience in his personal practice. Like many of the other authors of acumoxa literature, he was born into a family with a long history of medical practice, in his case in what is now the southeastern province of Zhèjiāng in 1522. His family's high social status is reflected in the fact that his grandfather held the position of imperial physician at court. In his family's extensive library of medical texts, Yáng was able to familiarize himself with the rich history of medical texts from an early age on. After he failed the imperial examinations for entering government service as a scholar-bureaucrat, he is said to have abandoned his studies of "Confucian medicine" and instead began an apprenticeship in his family. Fascinated with medical theory and diligent in gathering experience, he soon made a name for himself as an outstanding physician who excelled at both acupuncture/moxibustion and me-dicinal therapy. During the reign period Jiàng Qìng 降慶 (1567-1573), he entered service at the "Hall for Sagely Relief from Suffering," in other words, the imperial dispensary of the Míng court, where he gathered clinical experience until past the age of 50.

Aided by long years of personal experience and always with a focus on clinical applicability, he revised and annotated the major texts on acupuncture and moxibustion, which culminated in the compilation of the *Great Compendium of Acupuncture and Moxibustion* in 1601. Written in ten vol-umes with an extremely comprehensive content, this grand opus explains the theory and practice of acupuncture and moxibustion from a variety of angles, but always with an orientation toward clinical practice. Starting with a discussion on the sources of acupuncture and review of the theo-retical treatises from the *Inner Classic of the Yellow Emperor* and the *Classic of Difficult Issues* in volume one, volume two and three offer a selection of acupuncture-and moxibustion-related rhymed prose poems and songs. The subsequent volumes offer schematic charts of acumoxa point locations and channels, introduce the needling and moxibustion techniques of famous practitioners throughout history, discuss acumoxa in terms of its therapeutic significance and discuss technical details like the calendrical system based on the stems and branches, etc. Lastly, Yáng Jìzhōu included a selec-tion of his own case histories and a chapter on pediatric massage. Throughout the pages of this text, we find evidence of the author's personal experience in medicine, most notably in his fresh clinical approaches and the practical specifics presented in great detail.

This book greatly influenced the development of acupuncture and moxibustion after the Míng period in both China and Japan. As mentioned above, it also became the most important acumoxa text in Europe as well and was instrumental in generating a fascination with acupuncture in the French medical world due to the teaching and writing activities of George Soulie de Morant in the early twentieth century. Its lack of fame in the English-speaking world is most certainly not due to inadequacies in content but simply to the lack of an English-language translation. The present translation of the first volume of the *Great Compendium of Acupuncture and Moxibustion* is a true labor of love that has been produced with the intention and hope that it will be enjoyed and found

針灸大成 · 卷之一

useful by practitioners, students, and teachers of Chinese medicine who are unable to read it in the original Chinese. To fruitfully contemplate the information contained in this translation of the first volume of historical excerpts in particular, and to apply it meaningfully in the present, as it was certainly intended to be used by the author himself, rather than just reading it as an academic source with limited historical value, we must continuously bear the historical facets described above in mind.

For the sake of readability, ease of access, and clinical applicability, I have been forced to make some choices regarding terminology that have sometimes left me as an academically trained translator somewhat uncomfortable. I am grateful to my publisher, Jonathan Schell from the Chinese Medicine Database, and to Lorraine Wilcox, translator of volume five of the *Great Compendium*, for their willingness to engage in seemingly endless discussions on issues of translation and for sharing their clinical perspectives, which have undoubtedly made the text a more useful tool for the clinician. Foremost, and admittedly most contentious among these hard choices, was the decision to follow the modern convention of identifying acumoxa points not by their standard pīnyīn names (as has always been the convention in Chinese texts) nor by their English translations but by the combination of channel and number (i.e., Shén Cáng 神藏 (KI-25) Spirit Storehouse). Initially, I firmly resisted this change for three reasons: First, we lose so much information when we leave out the often-times highly expressive Chinese names, so full of historical, therapeutic, sensory, or other significance that, in my eyes, often contributes to an improved clinical understanding of the point and hence more effective use of the point in clinic. Second, as the discussion above has mentioned in fleeting, the acumoxa points originated in a very different textual and literary tradition (*yǎng shēng*, nurturing life primarily by sexual and breath cultivation) than the concept of the channel system (the so-called "acumoxa classics," addressing diseases in different regions of the body), which were only merged around the beginning of the Common Era at the earliest. And third, and perhaps most importantly, the numbered points instantly evoke in the modern reader's mind the anatomical charts and precise descriptions found in contemporary acupuncture textbooks. By contrast, a Chinese reader of the *Great Compendium* before the great systematization, standardization, and modernization that revolutionized Chinese medicine during the Communist Era beginning in the 1950s and before the arrival of X-ray and other modern biomedical imaging technology would have had a much vaguer, more intuitive and personalized approach to point localization, based on his or her clinical and sensory experience by means of nothing but touch and awareness of qì. Our understanding of ST-42 must have therefore been quite different from the associations assumed by Yáng Jìzhōu for chōngyáng 衝陽 or "Surging Yáng". Nevertheless, my colleagues have convinced me to adopt the system of identifying acumoxa point by associated channel and number because that is the way the points are learned and recognized by modern practitioners in English.

Moreover, as translator, I have chosen to consistently adopt Nigel Wiseman's standardized terminology for translating medical texts, as laid out in his *Practical Dictionary of Chinese Medicine*.[12] Even though the occasional awkward term—most notably the much-disputed use of "vacuity" and "repletion" instead of the more common "deficiency" and "excess" as translations for *xū* 虛 ("empty") and *shí* 實 ("full")—might initially throw the untrained reader off, the reason for this choice is simply that this terminology, when used in conjunction with Wiseman and Feng's dictionary, gives any reader with even limited skills in reading classical Chinese the tool to "read the text backwards," so to speak, and to know exactly which Chinese concept the English translation is referring to. Any instances where my choice of terminology deviates from Wiseman's terminology are specifically explained in the footnotes. It is my conviction that accuracy, consistency, and transparency are of utmost importance in the translation of any technical literature but especially of a medical text from seventeenth-century China. While an exact reproduction in a language as foreign as modern English is admittedly impossible, I have made every effort to avoid any culture-bound or personal interpretation of the material that might obscure the meaning of the original text. By following as literal a translation methodology as stylistic demands of the English language permit, what I might have sacrificed in elegance, I have gained in accuracy and faithfulness to the original source. As the reader, you may interpret the material as you wish, based on your particular combination of Chinese language skills and clinical experience in Chinese medicine.

It is my sincere hope as translator that by bringing this book to light in an environment so far removed in time, language, and culture, I will allow you, the reader, to also partake of the wisdom expressed in its lines and be inspired to search deeper in your own practice, both in the treatment of your patients and in the cultivation of your own physical, mental, and spiritual health in the spirit of *yǎng shēng* 養生.

---

12. Nigel Wiseman and Feng Ye, *A Practical Dictionary of Chinese Medicine*, second edition (Paradigm Publications, 1998). I am grateful to my friend and colleague Nigel Wiseman for countless discussions on the issue of translating Chinese medical literature with a standardized terminology, an issue that I was quite blissfully unaware of at the beginning of my career as a medical translator.

Acknowledgements

I dedicate this book to my dog Mr. Nilsson who has sustained me through countless months of brain-racking translation work by warming my feet under the desk and by greeting every break with excited tail-wagging. His exuberance reminds me every morning of how blessed I am to be living in such a beautiful universe.

Publisher's Note

In this series, the *Great Compendium of Acupuncture and Moxibustion,* the Chinese Medicine Database elected to use multiple translators to translate the different volumes. We did this so that our community would have access to the corpus of this text, sooner rather then later. There are many, many books that need to be translated, and if each translator did all of one large book, it would consume much of their life.

We have come to look at each volume as its own work, with each translator providing a slightly different, but similar voice to the translation. Everyone who has participated in this project has come to agreement that even though the same base translation dictionaries will be used, there is no way to produce a homogenous translation from one volume to the next. Expect to see small variations in reference to channel names like GV versus Du, as each translator uses the style that she feels the most comfortable with. I believe that the discrepancies are mostly topical, and I hope that the reader who has waited for years to the read the *Great Compendium*, will feel the same way.

There have been a number of sacrifices on the part of the translators to certain individual standards as the Database works out the best way to present this material. For example, we believe that inclusion of point numbers help modern readers understand the content of the classics better. We have appreciated the "team spirit" that everyone has shared in the project, and the willingness to work through difficult issues together.

仰人周身總穴圖
Chart of Major Points All Over the Body in the Supine Position

伏人周身總穴圖

Chart of Major Points All Over the Body in the Prone Position

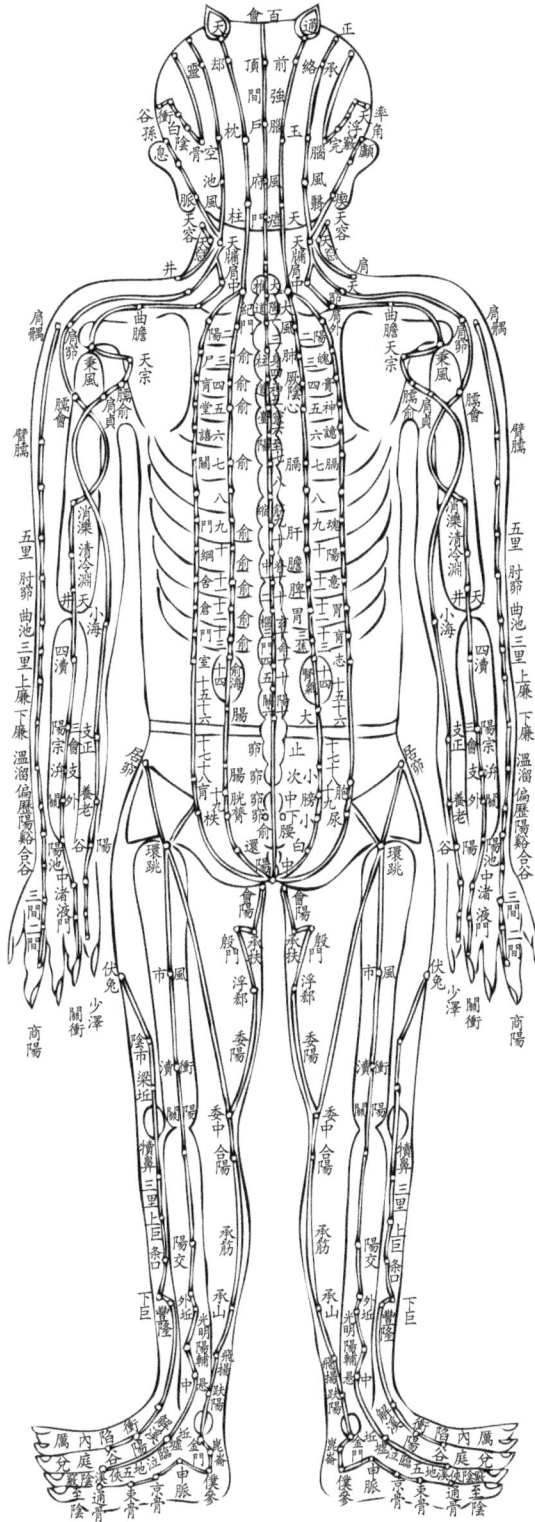

I. Direct Guide to Acupuncture and Moxibustion
Zhēn Jiǔ Zhí Zhǐ
針灸直指

I.1 On the Appropriateness of Acupuncture and Moxibustion According to Locality*
Zhēn jiǔ fāng yí lùn
針灸方宜論

Note:

* Excerpted from *Sù Wèn* 素問 (Plain Questions) 12, *Yì Fǎ Fāng Yí Lùn* 異法方宜論 (Treatise on the Appropriateness of Different Methods According to Locality).

Line 1

黃帝問曰：醫之治病也，一病而治各不同，皆愈何也？

The Yellow Emperor asked: Why is it that a physician when treating a single disease [in a number of patients] applies different treatments but all are cured?"

Line 2

岐伯對曰：地勢使然也。

Qíbó answered: "The forces of the land* are the reason for this.

Note:

* I have consciously chosen this somewhat clumsy translation of *dì shì* 地勢 because it is more literal than a phrase like "regional circumstances" or the modern "topography." My translation attempts to reproduce the significance of this term, which the famous Wáng Bīng 王冰, commentator of the *Huáng Dì Nèi Jīng* 黃帝內經 (Inner Classic of the Yellow Emperor) describes as follows: "Forces of the land refers to the dynamics/ forces that determine birth, growth, harvest, and storage, high and low locations, and dryness and dampness in heaven and on earth."

Line 3

(一)故東方之域，天地之所始生也，魚鹽之地，海濱傍水 。(二)其民食魚而嗜鹹，皆安其處，美其食 。(三)魚者使人熱中，鹽者勝血，故其民皆黑色疏理 。(四)其病皆為癰瘍 。(五)其治宜砭石，故砭石者，亦從東方來 。

(1) Thus, the region of the east[1] is the origin of heaven and earth, the land of fish and salt, of seashores and proximity to water. (2) Its people eat fish and crave salty foods, are settled in their places, and love their food. (3) Fish causes people to have heat in the center, and salt overcomes the blood.[2] Therefore, its people all have a black complexion and freely coursing interstices. (4) Their diseases are always welling abscesses and sores. (5) When treating here, it is appropriate to use wedge stones.[3] Wedge stones therefore also come from the East.

Notes:

1. This chapter is obviously based on the doctrine of the five phases and correlative thinking, which associates the five phases (wood, metal, water, fire, and earth) with the five direction (east, west, north, south, and center), the five seasons (spring, fall, winter, summer, and the intercalary month or late summer), etc. Hence the region of the East, for example, is associated with spring, wood, growth, and activity.
2. In traditional Chinese dietetics, fish is associated with fire, and excessive consumption of fish therefore causes heat to accumulate in the stomach. Similarly, salt is beneficial in moderate amounts, but damages the blood if consumed in excess.
3. *Biān shí* 砭石: This term describes the pointed stones that have been used traditionally for lancing and are one of the ancestors of traditional acupuncture.

Line 4

(一)西方者，金玉之域，沙石之處，天地之所收引也 。(二)其民陵居而多風，水土剛強。(三)其民不衣而褐薦，其民華食而脂肥，故邪不能傷其形體，其病生於內 。(四)其治宜毒藥，故毒藥者，亦從西方來 。

(1) The West is the region of gold and jade, the location of sand and stone, and the place where heaven and earth contract and draw inward.[1] (2) Its people reside [high up] in the mountains, there is a lot of wind, and the water and soil are hard and firm. (3) Its people do not wear fancy dresses and have only coarse woolen garments and straw mats. They have an extravagant diet and are fat. Therefore [external] evils cannot damage their physical bodies, and their diseases are generated internally. (4) When treating here, it is appropriate to use toxic medicinals.[2] Toxic medicinals therefore also come from the West.

Notes:

1. The West is associated with metal, autumn, the time of harvesting, and contraction. Toxic medicinals are appropriate here because they encourage drainage and elimination of waste.
2. Toxic medicinals here are to be understood in the sense of the lowest among the three categories of medicinals described in the *Shén Nóng Běn Cǎo Jīng* 神農本草經 (Divine Farmer's Classic of Materia Medica), i.e. medicinals that have the effect of moving and freeing qì and blood and thereby expelling evils.

Line 5

(一)北方者，天地所閉藏之域也 。(二)其地高陵居，風寒冰冽，其民樂野處而乳食 。(三)臟寒生滿病，其治宜灸焫，故灸焫者，亦從北方來 。

(1) The North is the region where heaven and earth close down and store. (2) Its land is high [in elevation] and the people live by the hills, with [a lot of] wind, cold, and ice. Its people like to spend time in the wild and consume dairy products. (3) Cold in the viscera engenders fullness disorders. When treating here, it is appropriate to use moxibustion.* Moxibustion therefore also comes from the North.

Note:

* It makes perfect intuitive sense that moxibustion is the suitable treatment for the
North, associated with water, winter, cold, and extreme yīn, especially since cold inhibits
the flow of blood and qì and therefore results in conditions associated with blockages
and repletion.

Line 6

(一)南方者，天地所長養，陽之所盛處也 。(二)其地下，水土弱，霧露之所
聚也 。(三)其民嗜酸而食胕，故其民皆致理而赤色 。(四)其病攣痹，其治宜
微針 。(五)故九針者，亦從南方來 。

(1) The South is where heaven and earth grow and nurture, the location where yáng
is exuberant. (2) Its land is low [in elevation], the water and soil are weak, and fog
and dew collect there. (3) Its people crave the sour flavor and eat fermented foods.
Therefore, they all have tight interstices and a red complexion. (4) Their diseases
are hypertonicity and impediment. When treating here, it is appropriate to use tiny
needles. (5) Therefore, nine needles therapy also comes from the South.

Line 7

(一)中央者，其地平以濕，天地所以生萬物也眾 。(二)其民食雜而不勞，故
其病多痿厥寒熱 。(三)其治宜導引按蹻，故導引按蹻者，亦從中央出也 。

(1) In the center, the land is level and damp, and for this reason heaven and earth can
bring forth a multitude of products. (2) Its people have a varied diet and do not over-
exert themselves. Therefore, their diseases tend to be wilting and reversal, [aversion
to] cold and heat [effusion]. (3) When treating here, it is appropriate to use guiding
and pulling, pressing and plucking.* Guiding and pulling and pressing and plucking
therefore also come from the center.

Note:

* These four terms refer to specific techniques of manual manipulation for the purpose
of qì-cultivation and promoting the free flow of qì and blood in the vessels, roughly
related to yoga-like stretching and massage, carried out either by the practitioner or the
patient him- or herself.

Line 8

(一)故聖人雜合以治，各得其所宜 。(二)故治所以異，而病皆愈者，得病之情，知治之大體也 。

(1) Hence the sage combines the various treatments, giving each [patient] what is appropriate for them. (2) The reason why treatments are different and yet the diseases are all cured is thus that the sage grasps the [specific] condition of the disease and know the general principle of therapy."

I.2 On Pricking[1] for Heat[2]
Cì rè lùn
刺熱論

Notes:

1. A note on translating *cì* 刺: Given how little we still know about the concrete implements used in the early history of acupuncture to manipulate qì and blood in the vessels, I have consciously chosen to translate this term as literally as possible, rather than using the more elegant modern translation of "needling." In my experience, when the early classics refer to the application of fine needles in the modern sense of tiny metal pins, they specifically refer to *zhēn* 針 ("needle") or even *wēi zhēn* 微針 ("fine needle"). I find the term "needle" as a translation of the broader *cì* potentially misleading to the modern reader, especially in contexts where the treatment involves bleeding the patient, sometimes to the point of drawing blood in drops the size of soybeans or until the blood changes color. See my note on translation in the introductory essay to this volume.
2. Excerpted from *Sù Wèn* 32, *Cì Rè* 刺热 (Pricking for Heat).

Line 1

黃帝問曰：五臟熱病奈何？

The Yellow Emperor asked: "How does heat disease [affect] the five viscera?"

Line 2

(一)岐伯曰：肝熱病者，小便先黃、腹痛、多臥、身熱。(二)熱爭則狂言及驚、脅滿痛、手足躁、不得安臥。(三)庚辛甚，甲乙大汗，氣逆則庚辛死。(四)刺足厥陰、少陽。(五)其逆則頭痛員員，脈引衝頭也。

(1) Qíbó answered: "The disease of liver heat presents first with yellow urine, abdominal pain, increased sleeping, and generalized heat [effusion]. (2) When the [evil qì of] heat struggles [with right qì], manic raving and fright, fullness and pain in the rib-side, agitated hands and feet, and inability to sleep soundly result. (3) On *gēng*

xīn days, the condition is aggravated; on *jiǎ yǐ* days, you will see great sweating.* Patients with qì counterflow will consequently die on a *gēng xīn* day. (4) Prick the foot juéyīn and shàoyáng vessels. (5) If [liver qì ascends] counterflow in these vessels, headache and dizziness result. This is the [heat] being drawn [upward in] the vessels and surging into the head.

Note:

> * *Gēng, xīn, jiǎ,* and *yǐ* are characters that designate days in the Chinese calendar. *Gēng xīn* is associated with metal, which can overcome wood (the liver is associated with wood). Thus liver disease worsens on these days. *Jiǎ yǐ* days are associated with wood. Because liver qì is effulgent on these days, right is able to overcome evil, hence we see great sweating and consequently lessened heat. For more information on the traditional Chinese calendar and the system for counting days, see Lorraine Wilcox's explanation in her translation of vol. 5 of the *Zhēn Jiǔ Dà Chéng,* published as *The Great Compendium of Acupuncture and Moxibustion Volume V,* The Chinese Medicine Database, 2010.

Line 3

(一)心熱病者，先不樂，數日乃熱 。(二)熱爭則卒心痛 、煩悶善嘔 、頭痛 、面赤無汗 。(三)壬癸甚，丙丁大汗，氣逆則壬癸死 。(四)刺手少陰 、太陽 。

(1) The disease of heart heat presents first with absence of joy. After a number of days, you will see heat. (2) When the [evil qì of] heat struggles [with right qì], sudden heart pain, vexation, oppression, and tendency to retch, headache, a red face, and absence of sweating result. (3) On *rén guǐ* days, the condition is aggravated; on *bǐng dīng* days, you will see great sweating. Patients with qì counterflow will consequently die on a *rén guǐ* day. (4) Prick the hand shàoyīn and tàiyáng vessels.

Line 4

(一)脾熱病者 、先頭重 、頰痛 、煩心 、顏青 、欲嘔 、身熱 。(二)熱爭則腰痛 、不可用俛仰 、腹滿泄 、兩頷痛 。(三)甲乙甚，戊己大汗 。氣逆則甲乙死 。(四)刺足太陰 、陽明 。

(1) The disease of spleen heat presents first with heaviness in the head, pain in the cheeks, vexation in the heart, a green-blue complexion, desire to retch, and generalized heat. (2) When the [evil qì of] heat struggles [with right qì], lumbar pain, inabil-

ity to bend forward or backward, abdominal fullness and diarrhea, and pain in both jaws result. (3) On *jiǎ yǐ* days, the condition is aggravated; on *wù jǐ* days, you will see great sweating. Patients with qì counterflow will consequently die on a *jiǎ yǐ* day. (4) Prick the foot tàiyīn and yángmíng vessels.

Line 5

（一）肺熱病者，先淅然厥、起毫毛、惡風寒、舌上黃、身熱。（二）熱爭則喘欬、痛走胸膺背、不得太息、頭痛不堪、汗出而寒。（三）丙丁甚，庚辛大汗。氣逆則丙丁死。（四）刺手太陰、陽明。（五）出血如大豆，立已。

(1) The disease of lung heat presents first with shivering, reversal, and raised body and head hair, aversion to wind and cold, yellow [fur] on the tongue, and generalized heat [effusion]. (2) When the [evil qì of] heat struggles [with right qì], panting and coughing; pain running into the chest, breasts, and back; inability to inhale deeply; unbearable headache, and sweating that is followed by [aversion to] cold result. (3) On *bǐng dīng* days, the condition is aggravated; on *gēng xīn* days, you will see great sweating. Patients with qì counterflow will subsequently die on a *bǐng dīng* day. (4) Prick the hand tàiyīn and yángmíng vessels. (5) Make the patient bleed with drops the size of soybeans, and recovery will ensue.

Line 6

（一）腎熱病者，先腰痛、胻痠、苦渴數飲、身熱。（二）熱爭則項痛而強、胻寒且痠、足下熱、不欲言。（三）其逆則項痛、員員澹澹然。（四）戊己甚，壬癸大汗，氣逆則戊己死。（五）刺足少陰、太陽。（六）諸汗者，至其所勝日汗出也。

(1) The disease of kidney heat presents first with lumbar pain and soreness in the calves, bitter thirst with frequent [desire to] drink, and generalized heat [effusion]. (2) When the [evil qì of] heat struggles [with right qì], pain and rigidity in the vertex of the head, cold as well as soreness in the calves, heat below the feet, and reluctance to speak result. (3) If [kidney qì] runs counterflow, pain in the nape of the neck, dizziness, and indifferent [behavior] result. (4) On *wù jǐ* days, the condition is aggravated; on *rén guǐ* days, you will see great sweating. Patients with qì counterflow will subsequently die on a *wù jǐ* day. (5) Prick the foot shàoyīn and tàiyáng vessels. (6) For all sweating, the sweat emerges when the day of overcoming arrives.[*]

Note:

> * In the treatment of heat conditions, the emergence of sweat signifies recovery because the heat is effused with the sweat. The "day of overcoming" (shèng rì 勝日) refers to the particular day associated with the phase of the viscus where the heat is located, because on this day the qì of the viscus is effulgent and therefore able to overcome the heat evil.

Line 7

(一)肝熱病者，左頰先赤 。(二)心熱病者，顏先赤 。(三)脾熱病者，鼻先赤 。(四)肺熱病者，右頰先赤 。(五)腎熱病者，頤先赤 。(六)病雖未發，見赤色者刺之，名曰治未病 。

(1) In liver heat disease, the left cheek turns red first. (2) In heart heat disease, the forehead turns red first. (3) In spleen heat disease, the nose turns red first. (4) In lung heat disease, the right cheek turns red first. (5) In kidney heat disease, the jaw turns red first. (6) Even though the disease has not yet emerged, if you see the red complexion, prick it. This is called "treating a disease before it arises."

Line 8

(一)熱病從部所起者，至期而已 。(二)其刺之反者，三周而已 。(三)重逆則死 。(四)諸當汗者，至其所勝日，汗大出也 。(五)諸治熱病，以飲之寒水，乃刺之 。(六)必寒衣之，居止寒處，身寒而止也 。

(1) If you address heat disease starting from the section [of the body/face] where it is located, the patient will recover when the time [for overcoming] arrives.[1] (2) If your pricking is contrary to this,[2] the patient will recover only after three cycles.[3] (3) If you go against [the correct therapy] yet again, death will result. (4) In all cases [of heat disorders], when the patient is supposed to sweat, wait until the day of overcoming [associated with the viscus where the heat is located] has arrived, and sweat will emerge profusely.[4] (5) In all cases of treating heat disease, give the patient cold water to drink, and prick only afterwards. (6) You must dress the patient so as to keep him or her cold and ensure that the dwelling is cold. When the body is cold, [the disease] stops.

Notes:

1. This refers to the "day of overcoming" mentioned above, i.e. the day associated with the affected organ, during which its qi is strong enough to overcome the evil by sweating it out, e.g. the *jiǎ yǐ* 甲乙 day for the liver. As mentioned above, this positive result manifests in great sweating.

2. I.e., if you treat the spleen when the patient suffers from liver disease, if you treat the kidney in cases of spleen disease, if you treat the heart in cases of kidney disease, if you treat the lung in cases of heart disease, and if you treat the liver in cases of lung disease. Alternatively, some scholars interpret this phrase a little more freely, reading it as "if you prick incorrectly," i.e. if you use draining when you should supplement....

3. Three cycles (*sān zhōu* 三周) means that the patient will suffer from this heat condition for three complete calendrical cycles before recovering on the date when the "day of overcoming" associated with the affected viscus arrives for the third time.

4. Indicating recovery because the heat is discharged via the sweat.

Line 9

(一) 熱病先胸脅痛 、手足躁 ，刺足少陽 ，補足太陰 。病甚者為五十九刺 。 (二) 熱病始手臂痛者 ，刺手陽明 、太陰 ，而汗出止 。 (三) 熱病始於頭首者 ，刺項太陽 ，而汗出止 。 (四) 熱病始於足脛者 ，刺足陽明 ，而汗出止 。 (五) 熱病先身重 、骨痛 、耳聾 、好暝 ，刺足少陰 。病甚為五十九刺 。 (六) 熱病先眩冒而熱 、胸脅滿 、刺足少陰 、少陽 。

(1) When heat disease manifests first with pain in the chest and rib-side and agitation in the hands and feet, prick the foot shàoyáng vessel and supplement the foot tàiyīn vessel.[1] If the disease is severe, apply the 59 prickings [technique].[2] (2) When heat disease begins with pain in the arms and back of the hands, prick the hand yángmíng and tàiyīn vessels. When the patient sweats, [the heat] will stop.[3] (3) When heat disease begins in the head, prick the tàiyáng points on the nape of the neck. When the patient sweats, [the heat] will stop. (4) When heat disease begins in the feet and shins, prick the foot yángmíng vessel. When the patient sweats, [the heat] will stop. (5) When heat disease manifests first with generalized heaviness, bone pain, deafness, and somnolence, prick the foot shàoyīn vessel. If the disease is severe, apply the 59 prickings [technique]. (6) When heat disease manifests first with veiling dizziness and then heat and fullness in the chest and rib-side, prick the foot shàoyīn and shàoyáng vessels.

Notes:

1. This dual approach has two purposes: draining heat in the yáng aspect and supporting the yīn aspect.

2. This refers to the 59 points used in the treatment of heat disease. See chapter I.14, p. 85, *Cì shuǐ rè xué lùn* 刺水熱穴論 "Treatise on Pricking Points for Water and Heat" below and *Sù Wèn* 61. According to Wáng Bīng's commentary, these points fall into five categories: points for dispersing and draining any heat evil that is ascending counterflow in the yángmíng vessels, points for draining heat evil from the chest, points for draining heat evil from the stomach, points for draining heat evil from the extremities, and points for draining heat evil from the five viscera.

3. Alternatively, this last phrase could be translated here and in the following lines as "and stop when the patient sweats."

Line 10

（一）太陽之脈，色榮顴骨，熱病也 。（二）榮未交[1]，曰今且得汗，待時而已 。（三）與厥陰脈爭見者，死期不過三日 。（四）其熱病內連腎 。

(1) [Heat in] the tàiyáng vessel manifest in a thriving complexion on the cheekbone. This is the sign of heat disease [in this vessel].[2] (2) If [the complexion on the cheekbone] is thriving and not yet perished, I say that if you can now make the patient sweat, he or she will recover as soon as the right time comes.[3] (3) If you also see struggle in the juéyīn vessel,[4] the time of death will be no more than three days away.[5] (4) The reason is that the heat disease has joined internally with the liver.

Notes:

1. According to commentary tradition, *jiāo* 交 should be read as *yāo* 夭 "to perish" in this context. "Perished complexion" is a phrase used to describe patients with critical conditions that are difficult to treat, because the disease has already moved from the surface to the interior of the body.

2. This symptom is due to the fact that a branch of the tàiyáng vessel runs into the cheekbone. According to Chinese commentators, a "thriving complexion" means a dark red color. According to the progression of disease first described in the *Shāng Hán Lùn* 傷寒論 (Treatise on Cold Damage), external evils advance from the outermost level of tàiyáng to the innermost level of juéyīn.

3. Most likely, this refers to the "day of overcoming" mentioned above, such as a *jiǎ yǐ* day in liver disease.

4. Most *Sù Wèn* commentators and modern translators suggest to replace juéyīn here with shàoyīn. Nevertheless, given the connection to the liver later in the sentence (since juéyīn is the vessel associated with the liver), I translate this line literally.

5. The combination of tàiyáng and juéyīn symptoms means that the patient is suffering from *liǎng gǎn* 两感 or "double contraction" of bowels and viscera, on the surface and in the interior. The condition is therefore much more serious and likely to result in death.

Line 11

(一)少陽之脈，色榮頰前，熱病也 。(二)榮未交，曰今且得汗，待時而已 。(三)與少陰脈爭見者，死期不過三日 。

(1) [Heat in] the shàoyáng vessel manifests in a thriving complexion in the front of the jaw. This is the sign of heat disease [in this vessel]. (2) If [the complexion in front of the jaw] is thriving and not yet perished, I say that if you can now make the patient sweat, he or she will recover as soon as the right time comes. (3) If you also see struggle in the shàoyīn vessel,* the time of death will be no more than three days away.

Note:

 * See Line 10 note 4 above. Similarly, many commentators here replace shàoyīn with juéyīn.

Line 12

(一)熱病氣穴，三椎下間主胸中熱；四椎下間主鬲中熱；五椎下間主肝熱；六椎下間主脾熱；七椎下間主腎熱 。(二)榮在骶也，項上三椎陷者中也 。(三)頰下逆顴為大瘕，下牙車為腹滿，顴後為脅痛，頰上者鬲上也 。

(1) Qì holes[1] for [treating] heat disease:
- below the third vertebra: governs heat in the center of the chest.
- below the fourth vertebra: governs heat in the center of the diaphragm.
- below the fifth vertebra: governs heat in the liver.
- below the sixth vertebra: governs heat in the spleen.
- below the seventh vertebra: governs heat in the kidney.
(2) [The points for treating heat in the] construction [aspect] are on the sacrum, as well as in the center of the depression below the three vertebrae on the nape of the

neck.[2] (3) If the [redness that signifies heat disease] ascends counterflow from below the jaws to the cheeks, this signifies "great conglomeration [diarrhea]." [Redness] that descends into the jawbones signifies abdominal fullness; [redness] behind the cheekbones signifies pain in the rib-side, and [redness] above the jaw signifies [disease] above the diaphragm."

Notes:

1. I.e., acupuncture points.
2. Commentators and translators are in disagreement on the meaning of this passage. The Japanese commentator Tanba no Motoyasu 丹波元簡 (1775-1810) even admits directly that the meaning of these two sentences is unclear. According to most scholars, the "center of the depression below the third vertebra of the neck" refers to Dà Zhuī 大椎 (GV-14).

I.3 On Pricking for Malaria*
Cì nüè lùn
刺瘧論

Note:

* Excerpted from *Sù Wèn* 36, *Cì Nüè* 刺瘧 (Pricking for Malaria).

Line 1

黃帝問曰：刺瘧奈何？

The Yellow Emperor asked: "How do you go about pricking for malaria?"*

Note:

* Concerning, "malaria," Wiseman defines the Chinese concept of this disorder as "a recurrent disease characterized by shivering, vigorous heat [effusion], and sweating and classically attributed to contraction of summerheat during the hot season, contact with mountain forest miasma, or contraction of cold damp. Malaria is explained as evil qì latent at midstage (half exterior and half interior)" (Wiseman, *Practical Dictionary*, p. 383).

Line 2

（一）岐伯對曰：足太陽之瘧令人腰痛頭重、寒從背起、先寒後熱熇熇暍暍然、熱止汗出。（二）難已。（三）刺郄中出血。

(1) Qíbó answered: "Malaria in the foot tàiyáng vessel causes people to suffer from lumbar pain and heaviness of the head; cold arising from the back; first [aversion to] cold, then heat [effusion] with intensely blazing force; and sweating after the heat [effusion] stops. (2) It is difficult to cure. (3) Prick Xī Zhōng,* drawing blood.

Note:

> * Most likely, an alternate name for Wěi Zhōng 委中 (BL-40), in the center of the horizontal line in the bend of the knee. It could, however, also simply be interpreted literally as the "middle of the cleft."

Line 3

(一)足少陽之瘧令人身體解㑊、寒不甚、熱不甚、惡見人、見人心惕惕然。(二)熱多，汗出甚。(三)刺足少陽。

(1) Malaria in the foot shàoyáng vessel causes people to suffer from fatigue and lack of strength; [aversion to] cold and heat [effusion], neither of which are too severe; and aversion to seeing people and apprehension when being seen by others. (2) Heat [effusion] predominates [over aversion to cold], and sweating is severe. (3) Prick the foot shàoyáng [vessel].

Line 4

(一)足陽明之瘧令人先寒洒淅洒淅、寒甚久乃熱、熱去汗出。(二)喜見日月光火氣乃快然。(三)刺足陽明跗上。

(1) Malaria in the foot yángmíng vessel causes people to suffer first from [aversion to] cold with great shivering, then after a long period of severe cold from heat [effusion], and after the heat has departed, from sweating. (2) Such patients like exposure to the light of the sun and moon and the qì of fire, which makes them happy.[1] (3) Prick the foot yángmíng vessel above the instep.[2]

Notes:

> 1. Usually, yángmíng signifies a predominance of qì and blood, and the presence of evil heat in this aspect would cause a strong aversion to fire and heat. In the present condition, though, the yángmíng vessel has contracted cold, a yīn evil, and the patient therefore has a liking for yáng and heat.
> 2. This refers to Chōng Yáng 衝陽 (ST-42).

Line 5

(一)足太陰之瘧令人不樂、好太息、不嗜食、多寒熱、汗出。(二)病至則善嘔，嘔已乃衰。(三)即取之。

(1) Malaria in the foot tàiyīn vessel causes people to suffer from joylessness, a tendency to deep sighing, no pleasure in eating, increased [aversion to] cold and heat [effusion], and sweating. (2) When the disease arrives, there is a tendency to vomiting, and after vomiting, [the malaria] recedes. (3) Promptly select [the foot tàiyīn points and prick them].

Line 6

(一)足少陰之瘧令人嘔吐甚、多寒熱、熱多寒少、欲閉戶牖而處。(二)其病難已。

(1) Malaria in the foot shàoyīn vessel causes people to suffer from severe vomiting; increased [aversion to] cold and heat [effusion], with the heat being stronger than the cold; and the desire to shut windows and doors and stay put. (2) This condition is difficult to cure.

Line 7

(一)足厥陰之瘧令人腰痛、少腹滿、小便不利、如癃狀、非癃也、數便、意恐懼、氣不足、腹中悒悒。(二)刺足厥陰。

(1) Malaria in the foot juéyīn vessel causes people to suffer from lumbar pain, fullness in the lesser abdomen, inhibited urination that resembles dribbling urinary block but is not dribbling urinary block but merely frequent urination, a fearful and timid will, insufficiency of qì, and abdominal distress. (2) Prick the foot juéyīn [vessel].

Line 8

(一)肺瘧者令人心寒，寒甚熱，熱間善驚，如有所見者 。(二)刺手太陰，陽明 。

(1) Lung malaria causes people to suffer from cold in the heart,* heat effusion when the cold becomes severe, and tendency to fright in between heat [episodes], as if they had seen something [startling]. (2) Prick the hand tàiyīn and yángmíng [vessels].

Note:

   * As Zhāng Jièbīn 張介賓 explains, the lung is the "canopy of the heart" (*xīn zhī gài yě* 心之蓋也). If cold evil overwhelms the lung, the patient therefore experiences a sensation of cold in the heart.

Line 9

(一)心瘧者令人煩心甚 、欲得清水，反寒多，不甚熱 。(二)刺手少陰 。

(1) Heart malaria causes people to suffer from severe vexation in the heart and desire to drink cool water, which reverses to turn into increased [aversion to] cold and not very severe heat [effusion].* (2) Prick the hand shàoyīn [vessel].

Note:

   * These two sets of symptoms appear to contradict each other but can be explained as follows: The internal heat causes the heat vexation and desire for cool drinks in the body's interior where yáng qì and heat evil have bound with each other and lie depressed, while the cold evil is expelled to the exterior, where it causes cold symptoms. Depending on how you translate *fǎn* 反, an alternative reading of this line would be: "Heart malaria causes people to suffer from severe vexation in the heart and desire to drink cool water [in the inside] but from increased [aversion to] cold and not very severe heat [effusion] on the outside."

針灸大成 · 卷之一

Line 10

（一）肝瘧者令人色蒼蒼然、太息、其狀若死者 。（二）刺足厥陰見血 。

(1) Lung malaria causes people to suffer from a very somber complexion, deep sighing, and a death-like appearance. (2) Prick the foot juéyīn [vessel] until you see blood.

Line 11

（一）脾瘧者令人寒、腹中痛、熱則腸中鳴、鳴已汗出 。（二）刺足太陰 。

(1) Spleen malaria causes people to suffer from [aversion to] cold, pain in the center of the abdomen, heat followed by grumbling in the intestines,* and sweating after the grumbling is over. (2) Prick the foot tàiyīn [vessel].

Note:

* The intestines make a grumbling noise because the heat evil moves spleen qì. As yáng qì is thrust to the outside, it causes sweating, which resolves the heat.

Line 12

（一）腎瘧者令人洒洒然、腰脊痛宛轉、大便難、目眴眴然、手足寒 。（二）刺足太陽、少陰 。

(1) Kidney malaria causes people to suffer from shivering, pain in the lumbus and spine [especially] when turning sides, difficulty defecating, dizzy vision, and cold in the hands and feet. (2) Prick the foot tàiyáng and shàoyīn [vessels].

Line 13

(一)胃瘧者令人疽病也 、善飢而不能食 、食而支滿腹大 。(二)刺足陽明，太陰橫脈出血 。

(1) Stomach malaria causes people to suffer from flat-abscesses, tendency to hunger but inability to eat, and eating resulting in propping fullness and an enlarged abdomen. (2) Prick the transverse [network] vessels of the foot yángmíng and tàiyīn vessels, drawing blood.*

Note:

* According to Zhāng Jièbīn, this is a reference to Shāng Qiū 商邱 (SP-5) on the transverse line in front of the inner ankle. One modern commentary explains this line as an instruction to prick the points Lì Duì 厲兌 (ST-45), Zú Sān Lǐ 足三里 (ST-36), and Jiě Xī 解谿 (ST-41), all on the foot yángmíng vessel, and then to prick the network vessel points of the foot tàiyīn vessel to draw blood.

Line 14

(一)瘧發身方熱，刺跗上動脈，開其孔，出其血，立寒 。(二)瘧方欲寒，刺手陽明 、太陰，足陽明 、太陰 。

(1) In malaria episodes, when the body is just turning hot, needle the moving vessel above the instep, opening up the hole and drawing blood from it. (2) This will make the patient cold.[1] In malaria episodes, when the patient is just about to turn cold, prick the hand yángmíng, hand tàiyīn, foot yángmíng, and foot tàiyīn [vessels].[2]

Notes:

1. Here, cold is not meant in the pathological sense, but in the sense of relieving the patient's heat.
2. Presumably also opening up the holes and drawing blood.

Line 15

（一）瘧脈滿大急，刺背俞，用中針傍五胠俞各一，適肥瘦出其血 。（二）瘧脈小實急，灸脛少陰，刺指井 。（三）瘧脈緩大虛，便用藥不宜用針 。

(1) When the pulse in malaria is full, large, and urgent, prick the transport points on the back. [Also,] use a medium-sized needle and insert it in each of the five points below the armpits on the side [of the back][1] once, drawing blood as suitable in accordance with the patient's fatness or thinness. (2) When the pulse in malaria is small, replete, and urgent, burn moxa on the shàoyīn [vessel] on the shin and prick the well [points] on the fingers and toes.[2] (3) When the pulse in malaria is moderate, large, and vacuous, then use medicinals. It is not suitable to use needles.

Notes:

1. According to modern commentators, this refers to the following points: Pò Hù 魄戶 (BL-42), Shén Táng 神堂 (BL-44), Hún Mén 魂門 (BL-47), Yì Shè 意舍 (BL-49), and Zhì Shì 志室 (BL-52).
2. According to some interpretations, this only refers to the toes.

Line 16

（一）凡治瘧，先發如食頃，乃可以治，過之則失時也 。（二）諸瘧而脈不見，刺十指間出血，血去必已 。（三）先視身之赤如小豆者，盡取之 。

(1) In all treatment for malaria, you can only treat it before it erupts by about the time span it takes to eat a meal. If you miss this [opportunity], you lose the time [to cure the disease]. (2) Whenever you do not see the pulse in malaria, prick the points between the ten digits,* drawing blood. As the blood is removed, [the disease] is invariably cured. (3) If you first see red spots on the body the size of mung beans, select all of those.

Note:

* Here, it is unclear whether the text is referring to toes and/or fingers.

Line 17

十二瘧者，其發各不同時，察其病形，以知其何脈之病也 。

The twelve types of malaria each develop at different times. Observe the specific form each condition takes to know which vessel is diseased.

Line 18

(一)先其發時，如食頃而刺之，一刺則衰，二刺則知，三刺則已 。(二)不已，刺舌下兩脈出血 。(三)不已，刺郄中盛經出血，又刺項以下俠脊者必已 。(四)舌下兩脈者，廉泉也 。

(1) Preceding an eruption of the disease by about the time it takes to eat a meal, prick [the patient]. One pricking weakens the disease. Two prickings produce noticeable results. Three prickings stop the disease. (2) If [the disease] is still not stopped, prick the two vessels below the tongue, drawing blood. (3) If it is still not stopped, prick the exuberant channel by Xī Zhōng, drawing blood. In addition, prick below the neck along the spine, and the patient invariably recovers. (4) The "two vessels below the tongue" refers to Lián Quán (CV-23).

Line 19

刺瘧者，必先問其病之所先發者，先刺之 。

When pricking for malaria, you must always ask the location where the malaria first erupted beforehand and then prick that location first.

Line 20

(一)先頭痛及重者，先刺頭上及兩額 、兩眉間出血 。(二)先項背痛者先刺之 。(三)先腰脊痛者，先刺郄中出血 。(四)先手臂痛者，先刺手少陰 、陽明十指間 。(五)先足脛痠痛者，先刺足陽明十指間出血 。

(1) If [the malaria began with] headache and a heavy head, first prick the top of the head and between the two sides of the forehead and the two eyebrows, drawing blood.* (2) If [the malaria began with] pain in the nape and neck, first prick there.

44

(3) If [the malaria began with] pain in the lumbus and spine, first prick Xī Zhōng, drawing blood. (4) If [the malaria began with] pain in the arms and hands, first prick the hand shàoyīn and yángmíng [vessels] between the ten fingers. (5) If [the malaria began with] soreness and pain in the feet and calves, first prick the foot yángmíng [vessel] between the ten toes, drawing blood.

Note:

  * According to the commentary, this refers to Shàng Xīng 上星 (GV-23) and Bǎi Huì 百會 (GV-20), to Xuán Lú 懸顱 (GB-5), and to Cuán Zhú 攢竹 (BL-2).

Line 21

(一)風瘧，瘧發則汗出惡風，刺三陽經背俞出血者 。(二)胻痠痛甚，按之不可名，曰胻髓病，以鑱針針絕骨，出血立已 。(三)身體小痛，刺至陰 。(四)諸陰之井，無出血，間日一刺 。(五)瘧不渴，間日而作，刺足太陽，渴而間日作，刺足少陽 。(六)溫瘧，汗不出，為五十九刺 。

(1) For wind malaria, [which manifests with] malaria attacks followed by sweating and aversion to wind, prick the back transport points of the three yáng channels, drawing blood. (2) Soreness in the shin with severe pain that is unspeakable when pressed is called "shin marrow disease." Use a chisel needle to needle[1] Jué Gǔ (GB-39); when you draw blood, the pain will stop. (3) For minor pain in the body, prick Zhì Yīn (BL-67). (4) When pricking any yīn well points, do not draw blood and [only] prick once every other day. (5) If malaria manifests with no thirst and episodes on alternate days, prick the foot tàiyáng [vessel]. If it manifests with thirst and episodes on alternate days, prick the foot shàoyáng [vessel]. (6) For warm malaria with no effusion of sweat, apply the 59 prickings [technique]."[2]

Notes:

  1. Chisel needle (chán zhēn 鑱針) is one of the nine kinds of needles used in traditional acupuncture. It refers to a needle with a sharp pointed tip in the shape of an arrow, used for superficial pricking of the body's surface, hence for conditions located in the skin layer.
  2. The 59 prickings (wǔ shí jiǔ cì 五十九刺) is a treatment method for severe heat disease first mentioned in Sù Wèn 32 on "Pricking for Heat." See chapter I.2 "On Pricking for Heat", line 9, note 2, p. 34 above for more information.

I.4 On Pricking for Cough[*]
Cì ké lùn
刺咳論

Note:

[*] Excerpted from *Sù Wèn* 38, *Ké lùn* 咳論 (On Cough).

Line 1

黃帝問曰：肺之令人咳何也？

The Yellow Emperor asked: "How is it that the lung causes people to cough?"

Line 2

岐伯對曰：五腑六臟，皆令人咳，非獨肺也 。

Qíbó answered: "The five viscera and six bowels all cause people to cough. It is not true that it is only the lung [that makes people cough]."[*]

Note:

[*] According to Zhāng Zhìcōng 張志聰, "The lung governs qì and resides in the highest location [of all the viscera]. It is where the hundred vessels assemble. While cough is a symptom of the lung, evil in the five viscera and six bowels can all ascend to the lung and cause cough." In other words, cough may be a sign of disease in the lung, but it can be caused originally by pathological change in any of the other viscera and bowels that has risen to affect the lung, impairing its function of effusion and downbearing. Alternatively, disease in the lung can over time also spread to the other viscera and bowels and cause signs of disease there.

Line 3

帝曰：願聞其狀 。

The Yellow Emperor said: "I would like to hear what [the different types of cough] look like."

Line 4

(一)曰：皮毛者，肺之合也 。皮毛先受邪氣，邪氣以從其合也 。(二)其寒飲食入胃，從肺脈上至於肺，則肺寒，肺寒則内外合邪因而客之，則為肺咳 。(三)五臟各以其時受病 。非其時，各傳以與之 。(四)人與天地相參，故五臟各以治時感於寒，則受病 。(五)微則為咳，甚者為泄，為痛 。

(1) [Qíbó] answered: "The skin and body hair are linked to the lung. The skin and body hair are the first [part of the body] to contract evil qì, and the evil qì follows where they are linked to.[1] (2) [Furthermore,] cold drinks and foods enter the stomach and rise upward along the lung vessel into the lung, causing cold in the lung. Lung cold then results in a combination of external and internal evil, which therefore settles in the lung. This means lung cough. (3) The five viscera each contract disease in the season associated [with them in correlative thinking].[2] When it is not the season [associated with the lung], each [of the other viscera] can pass [their disease] on to [the lung]. (4) Humans interact with Heaven and Earth. Therefore each of the five viscera will fall ill if they contract cold during the particular season when they rule. (5) In mild cases, this means cough. In serious cases, it means diarrhea and pain.

Notes:

1. I.e. the lung.
2. This means the season associated with each viscus in the five phases of correlative thinking, i.e. the liver contracts disease in the spring, the heart in the summer, the spleen in the late summer, the lung in the autumn, and the kidney in the winter.

Line 5

乘秋則肺先受邪；乘春則肝先受之；乘夏則心先受之；乘至陰則脾先受之；
乘冬則腎先受之 。

If [the cold evil] overwhelms [the body] in the autumn, the lung is the first to contract the evil. If [the evil] overwhelms [the body] in the spring, the liver is the first to
contract it. If [the evil] overwhelms [the body] in the summer, the heart is the first to
contract it. If [the evil] overwhelms [the body] in the arrival of yīn,* the spleen is the
first to contract it. If [the evil] overwhelms [the body] in the winter, the kidney is the
first to contract it."

Note:

   * I.e. the season of long summer.

Line 6

帝曰：何以異之？

The [Yellow] Emperor said: "How do you distinguish between these?"

Line 7

(一)曰：肺咳之狀，咳而喘，息有音，甚則唾血 。(二)心咳之狀，咳則心
痛，喉中介介如梗狀，甚則咽腫喉痹 。(三)肝咳之狀，咳則兩脅下痛，甚則
不可以轉，轉則兩胠下滿 。(四)脾咳之狀，咳則右胠下痛，陰陰引肩背，甚
則不可以動，動則咳劇 。(五)腎咳之狀，咳則腰背相引而痛，甚則咳涎 。

(1) [Qíbó] said: "Lung cough looks like this: cough with panting, noisy breathing,
and in serious cases ejection of blood. (2) Heart cough looks like this: cough resulting in heart pain, a feeling as if there were an obstruction in the throat, and in serious cases, a swollen pharynx and impediment in the larynx. (3) Liver cough looks
like this: cough resulting in pain below both rib-sides and in serious cases inability
to turn sides; if the patient does turn, this results in fullness below both flanks. (4)
Spleen cough looks like this: cough resulting in pain below the right flank and dull
pain stretching into the shoulders and back, and in serious cases inability to move;

if the patient does move, the cough is aggravated. (5) Kidney cough looks like this: cough resulting in tightness and pain between the lumbus and back, and in serious cases cough with drool."

Line 8

帝曰：六腑之咳奈何，安所受病 。

The [Yellow] Emperor said: "What about cough in the six bowels? How do they contract the disease?"

Line 9

曰：五臟之久咳，乃移於六腑 。

[Qíbó] said: "Enduring cough in the five viscera is [eventually] transmitted to the six bowels.

Line 10

（一）脾咳不已，則胃受之 。胃咳之狀，咳而嘔，嘔甚則長蟲出 。（二）肝咳不已，則膽受之 。膽咳之狀，咳嘔膽汁 。（三）肺咳不已，則大腸受之 。大腸咳狀，咳而遺矢 。（四）心咳不已，則小腸受之 。小腸咳狀，咳而失氣，氣與咳俱失 。（五）腎咳不已，則膀胱受之，膀胱咳狀，咳而遺溺 。（六）久咳不已，則三焦受之 。三焦咳狀，咳而腹滿，不欲食飲 。

(1) If spleen cough is not stopped, the stomach contracts it. Stomach cough looks like this: cough with vomiting, which in severe vomiting results in long worms coming out.[1] (2) If liver cough is not stopped, the gallbladder contracts it. Gallbladder cough looks like this: cough with vomiting of bile. (3) If lung cough is not stopped, the large intestine contracts it. Large intestine cough looks like this: cough with fecal incontinence. (4) If heart cough is not stopped, the small intestine contracts it. Small intestine cough looks like this: cough with loss of qì,[2] so that [the patient] breaks wind and coughs [at the same time]. (5) If kidney cough is not stopped, the bladder contracts it. Bladder cough looks like this: cough with enuresis. (6) If [a patient suffers from] enduring cough that is not stopped, the triple burner contracts it. Triple burner cough looks like this: cough with abdominal fullness and no desire to eat or drink.

Notes:

1. I.e. vomiting of roundworms?
2. I.e. flatulence.

Line 11

此皆聚於胃，關於肺，使人多涕唾，而面浮腫，氣逆也 。

In all of these conditions, [cold evil] can gather in the stomach, which is connected to the lung. This causes the patient to [suffer from] increased nasal mucus and spittle, puffy swelling in the face, and qì counterflow."

Line 12

帝曰：治之奈何？

The [Yellow] Emperor asked: "How do you treat [these conditions]?"

Line 13

岐伯曰：治臟者治其俞，治腑者治其合，浮腫者治其經 。

Qíbó said: "To treat the viscera, treat their transport points. To treat the bowels, treat their uniting points. To treat puffy swelling, treat their channels."

I.5 On Pricking for Lumbar Pain[*]
Cì yāo tòng lùn
刺腰痛論

Note:

[*] Excerpted from *Sù Wèn* 41, *Cì yāo tòng* 刺腰痛 (Pricking for Lumbar Pain).

Line 1

黃帝問曰：腰痛起於何脈，刺之奈何？

The Yellow Emperor asked: "Which vessel does lumbar pain arise in? And how do you go about pricking it?"

Line 2

（一）岐伯曰：足太陽脈令人腰痛，引項脊尻背如重狀 。（二）刺其郄中太陽正經，出血 。（三）春無見血 。

(1) Qíbó answered: "When the foot tàiyáng vessel causes a person to suffer from lumbar pain, [the pain] stretches to the nape, spine, and buttocks, and the back feels as if weighed down by a heavy object. (2) Prick the tàiyáng channel directly at Xī Zhōng, drawing blood. (3) In the spring, do not make blood appear.

Line 3

(一) 少陽令人腰痛，如以針刺其皮中，循循然不可以俛仰，不可以顧 。(二) 刺少陽成骨之端，出血 。(三) 成骨在膝外廉之骨獨起者 。(四) 夏無見血 。

(1) When the shàoyáng vessel causes a person to suffer from lumbar pain, the pain feels as if being pierced with needles through the skin. The patient is constantly unable to bend forward or backward and to turn and look around. (2) Prick the shàoyáng vessel at the edge of the shin bone,* drawing blood. (3) The shin bone is the place where the bone at the outer edge of the knee protrudes. (4) In the summer, do not make blood appear.

Note:

* In some commentaries, *chèng gǔ* 成骨 is paraphrased as *jìng gǔ* 脛骨. The point is equated with the modern point Yáng Líng Quán 陽陵泉 (GB-34).

Line 4

(一) 陽明令人腰痛，不可以顧，顧如有見者，善悲 。(二) 刺陽明於胻前，三 痏，上下和之出血 。(三) 秋無見血 。

(1) When the yángmíng vessel causes a person to suffer from lumbar pain, the patient is unable to turn and look around. If he or she does turn around to look back, they act as if they had seen an apparition, and they have a tendency to sorrow. (2) Prick the yángmíng vessel in front of the calf[1] three times[2] and harmonize above and below,[3] drawing blood. (3) In the fall, do not make blood appear.

Notes:

1. This refers to the modern point Zú Sān Lǐ 足三里 (ST-36).
2. The character *wěi* 痏 literally means "lesion," hence also the marks left behind after an acupuncture or moxibustion treatment. From there it has become a technical term in medical literature, used to refer to the number of needles inserted during a treatment session. Note that this does NOT mean to insert a certain number of needles one after the other in exactly the same spot, but to create a number of "lesions" as the result of inserting multiple needles right next to each other.

3. This somewhat unclear phrase has been disputed and explained by innumerable *Sù Wèn* commentators in different ways: It can either be read as "harmonize [this point] with those above and below," i.e. also prick the points above and below Zú Sān Lǐ 足三 里 (ST-36), or as "harmonize [the flow of qì and blood] in the upper and lower part of the body." The second interpretation makes more sense to me personally, but my literal translation above gives the reader the choice to make up his or her own mind.

Line 5

(一)足少陰令人腰痛，痛引脊內廉 。(二)刺少陰於內踝上，二痏 。(三)冬無 見血，出血太多，不可復也 。

(1) When the foot shàoyīn vessel causes a person to suffer from lumbar pain, the pain stretches to the inner edge of the spine. (2) Prick the shàoyīn vessel above the inner ankle[1] twice. In the winter,[2] do not make blood appear. (3) If the bleeding is excessive, the patient will be unable to recover.

Notes:

1. This refers to the modern point Fù Liū 復溜 (KI-7).
2. The parallel line in the *Sù Wèn* has *chūn* 春 (spring) here instead of winter.

Line 6

(一)厥陰之脈令人腰痛，腰中如張弓弩弦 。(二)刺厥陰之脈在腨踵魚腹之 外，循之累累然，乃刺之 。(三)其病令人善[1]言嘿嘿[2]然不慧 。(四)刺之三 痏 。

(1) When the juéyīn vessel causes a person to suffer from lumbar pain, there is a feeling in the lumbus as in arched-back rigidity. (2) Prick the juéyīn vessel on the outside of the fish-belly [-like protrusion] by the calf and the heel. When you find a place that feels like a string of pearls, prick there. (3) Disease [of the juéyīn vessel] causes a person to have a tendency to taciturnity and lack of intelligence. (4) Prick it three times.

Notes:

1. In a parallel version of this text in *Tài Sù* 30, the character *shàn* 善 is missing.
2. I am reading this as a textual error for *mò mò* 默默 (silently), because this is what all editions of *Sù Wèn* 41 have.

Line 7

(一)解脈令人腰痛，痛而引肩，目䀮䀮然，時遺溲 。(二)刺解脈，在膝筋肉分間，郄外廉之橫脈，出血 。(三)血變而止 。

(1) When the divided vessel* causes a person to suffer from lumbar pain, [it can manifest in] pain that stretches to the shoulders, blurred vision, and periodic urinary incontinence. (2) [In such cases,] prick the divided vessel at the knee in the space between the flesh and the sinew, in the horizontal vessel on the outer edge of Xī Zhōng, drawing blood. (3) When the blood changes [in color], stop.

Note:

* *Jiě mài* 解脈: This refers to the section of the foot tàiyáng bladder channel where it is divided into two branches, after it descends from the head to the back of the neck.

Line 8

(一)解脈令人腰痛，如引帶，常如折腰狀，善恐 。(二)刺解脈，在郄中結絡如黍米 。(三)刺之血射以黑，見赤血而已 。

(1) When the divided vessel causes a person to suffer from lumbar pain, [it can manifest in a feeling] as if being pulled by the belt and as if the waist were broken, [accompanied by] a tendency to fright. (2) [In such cases,] prick the divided vessel at Xī Zhōng where there is a bound network vessel like a millet grain. (3) Prick it until blood shoots out that is black. When you see red blood,* stop.

Note:

* I.e. when the color of the blood changes from black to red.

Line 9

（一）同陰之脈令人腰痛，痛如小錘鋸¹其中，怫然腫。（二）刺同陰之脈，在外踝上絕骨之端，為三痏。

(1) When the combined yīn vessel[2] causes a person to suffer from lumbar pain, the pain feels as if a small mallet[3] were lodged in the person's center,[4] and the person also suffers from fury and swelling.[5] (2) Prick the combined yīn vessel at the edge of the interrupted bone above the outer ankle[6] three times.

Notes:

1. In *Sù Wèn* 41, this character is written as 居, which makes more sense.
2. *Tóng yīn zhī mài* 同陰之脈: A branch network vessel of the foot shàoyáng vessel.
3. *Tài Sù* 30 has *zhēn* 針 (needle) here instead of *chuí* 錘 (mallet).
4. This could also mean "in the middle of the person's waist."
5. Most likely meaning that the person is in such a state of emotional upheaval that the network vessel is enlarged as a result.
6. In some modern commentaries, this point is identified with Yáng Fǔ 陽輔 (GB-38).

Line 10

（一）陽維之脈令人腰痛，痛上，怫然腫。（二）刺陽維之脈，脈與太陽合腨下間，去地一尺所。

(1) When the yáng linking vessel causes a person to suffer from lumbar pain, the pain ascends [along the vessel, which becomes] swollen from fury. (2) Prick the yáng linking vessel at the place where it meets the tàiyáng vessel below the calf, about one *chǐ* up from the ground.[1,2]

Notes:

1. I.e., the modern point Chéng Shān 承山 (BL-57).
2. One *chǐ* is equal to 30 cm or 11.81 inches.

Line 11

（一）衡絡之脈令人腰痛，不可以俯仰，仰則恐仆。（二）得之舉重傷腰，衡絡絕，惡血歸之。（三）刺之在郄陽，筋之間上郄數寸，衡居為二痏出血。

(1) When the transverse network vessel causes a person to suffer from lumbar pain, they are unable to bend forward and backward, and if they do bend backward, they are afraid of falling forward. (2) [This disorder] is contracted by lifting something heavy and thereby damaging the lumbus. The transverse network vessel is cut off, and malign blood returns to [the lumbus]. (3) Prick it at Xī Yáng (BL-39)[1] and several *cùn* above Xī Zhōng between the sinews.[2] Where the transverse [network vessel] is lodged, prick twice, drawing blood.

Notes:

1. Xī yáng 郄陽: According to Wáng Bīng, this point can be identified as Wěi Yáng 委陽 (BL-39), above and to the side of Xī Zhōng 郄中 (BL-40).
2. Again citing Wáng Bīng and accepted by the modern commentary tradition, this point is the modern point Yīn Mén 殷門 (BL-37), between the two sinews behind the knee.

Line 12

（一）會陰之脈令人腰痛，痛上漯漯然汗出，汗乾令人欲飲，飲已欲走。
（二）刺直陽之脈上三痏，在蹻上郄下五寸橫居，視其盛者出血。

(1) When the yīn meeting vessel[1] causes a person to suffer from lumbar pain, the pain rises, making the patient sweat in rivers. When the sweat has dried up, it causes the person to want to drink fluids and, after drinking, be restless. (2) Prick above the straight yáng vessel[2] three times, and prick above Yáng Qiāo (BL-62) and below Xī Zhōng, five *cùn* from each, where the transverse [network vessel] is lodged and you can see it filled [with blood].[3] Draw blood.

Notes:

1. According to Wáng Bīng, this refers to the section of the foot tàiyáng vessel where its two branches meet at the anus below the lumbus (in Chinese called *hòu yīn* 後陰, "posterior yīn").

2. This refers to the straight section of the foot tàiyáng vessel in the leg. According to Wáng Bīng, this is the straight section behind the outer ankle after passing through the calves.

3. Most commentaries agree that this refers to Chéng Jīn 承筋 (BL-56).

Line 13

(一) 飛揚之脈令人腰痛，痛上怫怫然，甚則悲以恐 。(二) 刺飛揚之脈，在踝上五寸，少陰之前，與陰維之會 。

(1) When the Fēi Yáng [network] vessel* causes a person to suffer from lumbar pain, the pain rises, making the person furious. When it is severe, it results in sorrow and then fear. (2) Prick the Fēi Yáng [network] vessel five *cùn* above the ankle, anterior to the shàoyīn [vessel] and where it meets the yīn linking [vessel].

Note:

> * This refers to a small network vessel of the foot tàiyáng vessel, presumably in the vicinity of the Fēi Yáng 飛揚 point (BL-58).

Line 14

(一) 昌陽之脈令人腰痛，痛引膺，目䀮䀮然，甚則反折，舌卷不能言 。
(二) 刺內筋為二痏，在內踝上大筋前、太陰後上踝二寸所 。

(1) When the Chāng Yáng [network] vessel[1] causes a person to suffer from lumbar pain, the pain stretches to the breasts and the vision is unclear. If the condition is severe, it will result in arched-back [lumbus and lower back],[2] and in a curled tongue and inability to speak. (2) Prick twice at the inner sinew, above the inner ankle in front of the large sinew, two *cùn* above the ankle behind the tàiyīn vessel.[3]

Notes:

> 1. This most likely refers either to Fù Liū 復溜 (KI-7) itself or to a small network vessel of the foot shàoyīn kidney channel in the vicinity of Fù Liū (KI-7).
>
> 2. This phrase has clear associations with the dreaded disease *jiǎo gōng fǎn zhāng* 角弓反张 ("arched-back rigidity"), which is frequently called *yāo fǎn zhé* 腰反折 ("arched-back lumbus").

3. Most likely a reference to Fù Liū 復溜 (KI-7).

Line 15

(一) 散脈令人腰痛而熱，熱甚生煩，腰下如有橫木居其中，甚則遺溲 。
(二) 刺散脈，在膝前骨肉分間，絡外廉束脈為三痏 。

(1) When the Sàn Mài [network vessel][1] causes a person to suffer from lumbar pain and heat, if the heat is severe, it engenders vexation and a feeling below the lumbus as if there were a tree lodged transversely in the person's center. In severe cases, it results in urinary incontinence. (2) Prick the Sàn Mài [network vessel] in front of the knee at the seam between the flesh and the bone, on the vessel that is bundling the network vessels on the exterior edge,[2] three times.

Notes:

1. Literally translated as "scattered vessel," this term refers to a small network vessel of the foot tàiyīn vessel in the lower leg.
2. According to modern commentary tradition, this is a reference to Dì Jī 地機 (SP-8).

Line 16

(一) 肉里之脈，令人腰痛不可以欬，欬則筋縮 。(二) 刺肉里之脈為二痏，在太陽之外，少陽絕骨之後 。

(1) When the Ròu Lǐ [network] vessel[1] causes a person to suffer from lumbar pain, [the pain is so severe that] the person is unable to cough, and if they do cough, it makes the sinews contract. (2) Prick the Ròu Lǐ [network] vessel twice, on the outside of the tàiyáng [vessel] and in the back of Jué Gǔ (GB-39)[2] on the shàoyáng [vessel].

Notes:

1. Lit., "flesh pattern." A branch network vessel that originates from the foot shàoyáng vessel in the lower leg.
2. Lit. "interrupted bone," an alternate name for Xuán Zhōng 懸鐘 (GB-39).

Line 17

（一）腰痛俠脊而痛，至頭幾幾然，目䀮䀮，欲僵仆，刺足太陽郄中出血 。
（二）腰痛上寒，刺足太陽陽明 。（三）上熱，刺足厥陰 。（四）不可以俯仰，刺
足少陽 。（五）中熱而喘，刺足少陰，刺郄中出血 。（六）腰痛上寒不可顧，刺
足陽明 。（七）上熱，刺足太陰 。（八）中熱而喘，刺足少陰 。（九）大便難，刺
足少陰 。（十）少腹滿，刺足厥陰 。（十一）如折不可以俛仰，不可舉，刺足
太陽 。（十二）引脊內廉，刺足少陰 。（十三）腰痛引少腹控䏚，不可以仰，
刺腰尻交者，兩髁胂上 。

(1) For lumbar pain that pinches the the spine and ascends into the head, [causing] discomfort in the neck,[1] blurred vision, and verging on sudden collapse, prick Xī Zhōng on the foot tàiyáng [vessel], drawing blood. (2) For lumbar pain with [aversion to] cold in the upper body, prick the foot tàiyáng and yángmíng [vessels].[2] (3) [For lumbar pain with] heat [effusion] in the upper body, prick the foot juéyīn [vessel]. (4) [For lumbar pain with] inability to bend forward and backward, prick the foot shàoyáng [vessel]. (5) [For lumbar pain with] heat strike and panting, prick the foot shàoyīn [vessel]. Prick Xī Zhōng, drawing blood. (6) For lumbar pain with [aversion to] cold in the upper body and inability to turn to look around, prick the foot yángmíng [vessel]. (7) [For lumbar pain with] heat [effusion] in the upper body, prick the foot tàiyīn [vessel]. (8) [For lumbar pain] with heat strike and panting, prick the foot shàoyīn [vessel]. (9) [For lumbar pain] with difficult defecation, prick the foot shàoyīn [vessel]. (10) [For lumbar pain with] fullness in the lesser abdomen, prick the foot juéyīn [vessel]. (11) For a feeling as if [the lumbus] were broken, inability to bend forward and backward, and inability to lift,[3] prick the foot tàiyáng [vessel]. (12) [For lumbar pain] stretching to the inner edge of the spine, prick the foot shàoyīn [vessel]. (13) For lumbar pain stretching to the lesser abdomen and the empty space below the rib-sides, in conjunction with inability to bend backwards, prick the meeting point at the lumbus and coccyx,[4] on the buttocks above the coccyx.

Notes:

1. The literal meaning of the character *shū* 幾 describes a feeling like a bird with short wings and a stretched-out neck, trying to but being unable to fly.
2. This line and the following three lines up to "Prick Xī Zhōng, drawing blood" are not found in some editions of *Sù Wèn* 41. While this section contradicts or repeats information found in the following lines, I have chosen to retain it to give the reader an accurate idea of the original text.
3. I have translated this literally because the text is ambiguous here. It could mean "lift anything" or "raise the upper body."

4. According to Wáng Bīng, this refers to the area of the "eight bone holes" *bā liáo* 八髎 behind the sacrum to both sides of the coccyx. Since this is where the foot tàiyīn, juéyīn, and shàoyáng vessels meet, it is called the "meeting point at the lumbus and coccyx."

Line 18

（一）以月生死為痏數，發針立已 。（二）左取右；右取左 。

(1) Calculate the number of prickings by the waxing and waning of the moon, apply the needle, and that is all. (2) For [pain in the] left [side of the body], select the right [side of the body to apply treatment], for [pain in the] right [side of the body], select the left [side to apply treatment]."*

Note:

* The reason for this advice is that the vessels cross over to the other side of the body by the coccyx.

I.6 On Rare Diseases[1, 2]
Qí bìng lùn
奇病論

Notes:

1. Excerpted from *Sù Wèn* 47, *Qí bìng lùn* 奇病論 (On Rare Diseases).
2. At the very beginning of the text, there is a missing line from the *Sù Wèn*: The Yellow Emperor asked: "Why is it that [some] women who are pregnant lose their voice in the ninth month?" In the rest of this chapter, I have only marked major omissions that are important for content. I have paraphrased the *Sù Wèn* text in the footnotes.

Line 1

(一)岐伯曰：人有重身，九月而瘖，名曰胞之絡脈絕也 。(二)無治，當十月復 。

(1) Qíbó said: "When a woman who is pregnant loses her voice in the ninth month, this is called 'interrupted network vessels of the uterus.'[1] (2) Do not treat her. She will recover in the tenth month.[2]

Notes:

1. Following this line, *Sù Wèn* 47 offers additional information that is not repeated here. To paraphrase, the uterine network vessels are tied to the kidney and the shàoyīn vessel and thereby also to the root of the tongue. Hence the symptom of inability to speak.
2. Quoting the *Cì fǎ* 刺法 (Method of Needling), *Sù Wèn* 47 continues here with the warning not to treat insufficiency by reducing or to treat excess by boosting, thereby creating new complications.

Line 2

(一)病脅下滿氣逆，二三歲不已，名曰息積 。(二)不可灸刺，為導引服藥 。

(1) When a person suffers from fullness below the rib-side and qì counterflow that does not stop for 2 to 3 years, this is called 'breath accumulation.' (2) [This condition] cannot be treated with moxibustion or pricking, but with guiding and pulling and by ingesting medicine.*

Note:

> * Additional text in *Sù Wèn* 47 clarifies that you must first course the qì by guiding and pulling and cannot treat it with medicinals alone.

Line 3

(一)人身體髀股胻皆腫，環臍而痛，名曰伏梁 。(二)不可動之 。(三)動之為水溺濇之病也 。

(1) When a patient suffers from generalized swelling in the buttocks, upper, and lower leg and from pain encircling the navel, this is called 'deep-lying beam.'[1] (2) It cannot be treated by moving it.[2] (3) Moving it causes the disease of inhibited urination.

Notes:

> 1. *Sù Wèn* 47 elaborates that this condition is rooted in wind. When it spills into the large intestine and from there into the area below the navel, it causes pain there.
> 2. This is a warning against using aggressive treatment methods to eliminate the wind, such as "offensive precipitation" (*gōng xià* 攻下), i.e., prescribing toxic medicinals for draining, which would disturb bowel qì. The consequence of this incorrect treatment is explained in the next line.

針灸大成・卷之一

Line 4

（一）人有尺脈數甚，筋急而見，名曰疹筋。（二）是人腹必急。（三）白色黑色見，則病甚。

(1) When a person has an extremely rapid cubit (*chǐ*) pulse and sinews that are tense and visible, it is called 'diseased sinews.' (2) Such a person's abdomen is invariably tense. (3) When a white or black facial complexion is apparent, the disease is serious.

Line 5

（一）人有病頭痛，數歲不已，名曰厥逆。（二）謂所犯大寒，內至骨髓。（三）髓以腦為主，腦逆，故令頭痛，齒亦痛。

(1) When a person suffers from headache that persists for several years without stopping, it is called 'reverse flow.' (2) It is said that this is due to an invasion of great cold, which internally has arrived in the marrow of the bones. (3) Given the fact that the brain is the ruler of the marrow, it results in counterflow in the brain, which therefore causes headache and also toothache.

Line 6

（一）有病口甘者，名曰脾癉。（二）謂人數食甘美而多肥。肥者令人內熱，甘者令人中滿。（三）故氣上溢，轉為消渴。（四）治之以蘭，除陳氣也。

(1) There is a disease [that manifests with] sweetness in the mouth. It is called spleen *dàn*.[1] (2) It is said that this is due to people frequently eating sweet and rich foods and excessive fat. The fat causes internal heat in the person, while the sweets cause fullness in the center. (3) Therefore qì rises up and spills over, transforming into dispersion thirst.[2] (4) Treat it with orchid to eliminate the stale qì.

Notes:

1. Wiseman translates *dàn* 癉 as "pure heat," most commonly in the compound *dàn nuè* 癉瘧, pure-heat malaria. This translation stresses its heat-related etiology.
2. This disease is characterized by thirst, increased appetite, and copious urination, often associated with the modern biomedical disease category of diabetes.

Line 7

(一)有病口苦者，名曰膽癉 。(二)治之以膽募俞 。

(1) There is a disease [that manifests with] bitterness in the mouth. It is called gall-bladder *dàn*. (2) Treat it at the gallbladder alarm and transport points.

Line 8

(一)有癃者，日數十溲，此不足也 。(二)身熱如炭 、頸膺如格 、人迎躁盛 、喘息 、氣逆，此有餘也 。(三)太陰脈細微如髮者，此不足也 。(四)五有餘，二不足，名曰厥 。(五)死不治 。

(1) There is the disease of dribbling urinary block, in which [the patient] urinates several dozen times a day. This is [a sign of] insufficiency.[1] (2) Generalized heat [effusion] like roasting, a feeling like repulsion between the neck and chest, an agitated and exuberant pulse at Rén Yíng (ST-9), panting, and qì counterflow are [signs of] excess. (3) A tàiyīn pulse that is fine and faint like hair is [a sign of] insufficiency. (4) With the five [signs of] excess and the two [signs of] insufficiency,[2] this is called reversal. (5) The patient will die because [this disease] is untreatable.

Notes:

1. I.e., insufficiency of right qì. Similarly, the "excess" referred to in the next line means excess of evil qì.
2. This is a reference to the symptoms described in the previous lines. As the text in *Sù Wèn* 47 explains, given the fact that this disease combines five symptoms of excess on the exterior and two symptoms of insufficiency in the interior, you can neither treat it on the exterior nor in the interior, making it particularly difficult to treat.

Line 9

(一)人初生病癲疾者，名曰胎癇 。(二)謂在母腹中感驚，令子發為癲也 。

(1) When a baby right at birth suffers from withdrawal, this is called "fetal epilepsy." (2) It is said that [the fetus] contracted fright inside the mother's belly, which is causing episodes of epilepsy in the child.

針灸大成 • 卷之一

Line 10

(一)有病痝然，如有水狀、切其脈大緊、身無痛者、形不瘦、不能食、食少，名曰腎風。(二)腎風而不能食、善驚、驚已，心氣痿者死。

(1) There is a disease [that manifests] in swelling, an appearance as if water were present, a large tight pulse when palpated, no pain in the body, no emaciation, and inability to eat or eating very little. It is called kidney wind. (2) Kidney wind results in inability to eat, tendency to fright, and death from heart qì wilting when the fright stops.

Line 11

(一)有病怒狂者，名曰陽厥。(二)謂陽氣因暴折而難決，故善怒也。(三)治之當奪其食，即已，使之服以生鐵洛為飲。

(1) There is a disease that manifests in anger and mania. It is called yáng reversal. (2) It is said that the patient has difficulty deciding because yáng qì suddenly changes direction. Hence there is a tendency to anger. (3) To treat it, take away [the patient's] food and it will stop. Make [the patient] ingest iron flakes in a beverage.

Line 12

夫生鐵洛者，下氣疾也。

Iron flakes precipitate qì disease."

I.7 On the Essentials of Pricking[*]
Cì yào lùn
刺要論

Note:

[*] Excerpted from *Sù Wèn* 50, *Cì yào lùn* 刺要論 (On the Essentials of Pricking).

Line 1

黃帝問曰：願聞刺要 。

The Yellow Emperor asked: "I would like to hear about the essentials of pricking."

Line 2

(一)岐伯對曰：病有浮沉，刺有淺深，各至其理，無過其道 。(二)過之則內傷 。(三)不及則生外壅，壅則邪從之 。(四)淺深不得，反為大賊，內動五臟，後生大病 。(五)故曰病有在毫毛腠理者，有在皮膚者，有在肌肉者，有在脈者，有在筋者，有在骨者，有在隨者 。

(1) Qíbó replied: "There are superficial diseases and there are deep-lying ones.[1] There is shallow pricking and there is deep pricking. In each case, proceed to its pattern[2] but do not go beyond its pathway. (2) If you go beyond it, internal damage results. (3) If you do not reach far enough, you engender external congestion, and if there is congestion, the evil can follow it there. (4) If the [correct] depth [of pricking] is not achieved, you on the contrary cause major harm and internally stir the five viscera. Afterwards you generate serious illness. (5) Therefore I say that among diseases, some are located in the fine body hair and interstices, some in the skin, some in the flesh, some in the vessels, some in the sinews, some in the bones, and some in the marrow.

針灸大成・卷之一

Notes:

1. In other words, diseases of the exterior and of the interior.
2. Literally, *li* 理 means the veins in jade or the grain in wood, from which I derive the translation "pattern." Here, I interpret it as the specific layer in the body where the disease is located. Paul U. Unschuld uses the word "structure" here to convey this meaning, but 理 here also refers to non-structural entities, specifically the channels and network vessels. See his *Huang Di Nei Jing Su Wen: Nature, Knowledge, Imagery in an Ancient Chinese Medical Text* (University of California, 2003), p. 281. Modern Chinese editions simply paraphrase the sentence as "reach the specific location of the disease." I read it as a reference to the line below about disease being located in the body hair and interstices, skin, flesh, vessels, sinews, bones, or marrow.

Line 3

（一）是故刺毫毛腠理者，無傷皮 。（二）皮傷內動肺，肺動則秋病溫瘧，淅淅然寒慄 。

(1) For this reason, when pricking the fine body hair and interstices, do not damage the skin. (2) If the skin is damaged, this stirs the lung internally, and if the lung is stirred, the patient will suffer from warm malaria with shivering and cold shudders in the autumn.

Line 4

（一）刺皮，無傷肉 。（二）肉傷則內動脾，脾動則七十二日四季之月，病腹脹，煩不嗜食 。

(1) When pricking the skin, do not damage the flesh. (2) If the flesh is damaged, this stirs the spleen internally, and if the spleen is stirred, the patient will suffer from abdominal distention, vexation, and lack of appetite during the 72 days of the intercalary months.*

Note:

* This refers to the last 18 days of each season.

Line 5

(一)刺肉，無傷脈 。(二)脈傷則内動心，心動則夏病心痛 。

(1) When pricking the flesh, do not damage the vessels. (2) If the vessels are damaged, this stirs the heart internally, and if the heart is stirred, the patient will suffer from heart pain in the summer.

Line 6

(一)刺脈，無傷筋 。(二)筋傷則内動肝，肝動則春病熱而筋弛 。

(1) When pricking the vessels, do not damage the sinews. (2) If the sinews are damaged, this stirs the liver internally, and if the liver is stirred, the patient will suffer from heat [effusion] and slack sinews in the spring.

Line 7

(一)刺筋，無傷骨 。(二)骨傷則内動腎，腎動則冬病脹，腰痛 。

(1) When pricking the sinews, do not damage the bones. (2) If the bones are damaged, this stirs the kidney internally, and if the kidney is stirred, the patient will suffer from distention and lumbar pain in the winter.

Line 8

(一)刺骨，無傷髓 。(二)髓傷則銷鑠胻痠，體解㑊然不去矣 。

(1) When pricking the bones, do not damage the sinews. (2) If the sinews are damaged, the patient will suffer from the frailness of a chronic illness, soreness in the calves, sluggishness and fatigue, and inability to move around."

I.8 On the Level of Pricking[*]
Cì qí lùn
刺齊論

Note:

* Excerpted from *Sù Wèn* 51, *Cì qí lùn* 刺齊論 (On the Level of Pricking).

Line 1

黃帝問曰：願聞刺淺深之分 。

The Yellow Emperor asked: "I would like to hear about the difference between shallowness and depth in pricking."

Line 2

(一)岐伯曰：刺骨無傷筋者，針至筋而去，不及骨也 。(二)刺筋無傷肉者，至肉而去，不及筋也 。(三)刺肉無傷脈者，至脈而去，不及肉也 。(四)刺脈無傷皮者，至皮而去，不及脈也 。

(1) Qíbó said: "The warning against damaging the sinews when pricking the bones means that if the needle reaches only the sinews and is removed [without going deeper], it fails to reach the bones.[*] (2) The warning against damaging the flesh when pricking the sinews means that if [the needle] reaches the flesh and is removed, it fails to reach the sinews. (3) The warning against damaging the vessels when pricking the flesh means that if [the needle] reaches the vessels and is removed, it fails to reach the flesh. (4) The warning against damaging the skin when pricking the vessels means that if [the needle] reaches the skin and is removed, it fails to reach the vessels.

Note:

> * In other words, the practitioner has pricked too shallowly and therefore failed to reach the location of the disease, in this case the bones. In contrast to the previous chapter, this line is thus a warning against applying the needle too shallowly. The original *Sù Wèn* text starts with a list of warnings against pricking both too shallowly and too deeply in each of the five levels, namely the bones, sinews, flesh, vessels, and skin, progressing from the deepest to the shallowest level.

Line 3

(一)所謂刺皮無傷肉者，病在皮中，針入皮中，無傷肉也 。(二)刺肉無傷筋者，過肉中筋也 。(三)刺筋無傷骨者，過筋中骨也 。(四)此謂之反也 。

(1) What I mean by warning against damaging the flesh when pricking the skin is that the disease is in the skin and the needle should enter the skin instead of damaging the flesh. (2) The warning against damaging the sinews when pricking the flesh refers to going beyond the flesh and hitting the sinews. (3) The warning against damaging the bones when pricking the sinews refers to going beyond the sinews and hitting the bones. (4) This is what is called doing the opposite [of what is correct]."

I.9 On What to Bear in Mind During Pricking*
Cì zhì lùn
刺志論

Note:

    * Excerpted from *Sù Wèn* 53, *Cì zhì lùn* 刺志論 (On What to Bear in Mind During Pricking).

Line 1

黃帝問曰：顧聞虛實之要 。

The Yellow Emperor asked: "I would like to hear about the essentials of vacuity and repletion."

Line 2

(一)岐伯對曰：氣實形實，氣虛形虛 。(二)此其常也 。反此者病 。(三)穀盛氣盛，穀虛氣虛 。(四)此其常也 。反此者病 。(五)脈實血實，脈虛血虛 。(六)此其常也 。反此者病 。

(1) Qíbó answered: "When qì is replete, the body is replete. When qì is vacuous, the body is vacuous. (2) This is the normal state [of health]. The opposite of this is disease. (3) When the food intake* is plentiful, qì is plentiful. When the food intake is vacuous, qì is vacuous. (4) This is the normal state [of health]. The opposite of this is disease. (5) When the pulse is replete, the blood is replete. When the pulse is vacuous, the blood is vacuous. (6) This is the normal state [of health]. The opposite of this is disease."

Note:

    * Literally, "grains," a term that is commonly used to refer to diet in general.

71

Line 3

帝曰：如何而反？

The [Yellow] Emperor said: "What do you mean by 'opposite'?"

Line 4

(一)岐伯曰：氣虛身熱，此謂反也 。(二)穀入多而氣少，此謂反也 。(三)穀不入而氣多，此謂反也 。(四)脈盛血少，此謂反也 。(五)脈小血多，此謂反也 。

(1) Qíbó said: "When qì is vacuous but the body is hot, this is called opposite. (2) When the food intake is profuse but qì is scant, this is called opposite. (3) When there is no food intake but the qì is profuse, this is called opposite. (4) When the pulse is exuberant but the blood is scant, this is called opposite. (5) When the pulse is small but the blood is profuse, this is called opposite.

Line 5

(一)氣盛身寒，得之傷寒 。(二)氣虛身熱，得之傷暑 。(三)穀入多而氣少者，得之有所脫血，濕居下也 。(四)穀入少而氣多者，邪在胃及與肺也 。(五)脈小血多者，飲中熱也 。(六)脈大血少者，脈有風氣，水漿不入 。(七)此之謂也 。

(1) Qì exuberance with generalized cold is contracted as a result of cold damage. (2) Qì vacuity with generalized heat is contracted as a result of summerheat damage. (3) Profuse food intake with shortage of qì is contracted as a result of blood desertion and dampness lodged in the lower body. (4) Reduced food intake with profuse qì is the result of evil located in the stomach and lung. (5) A small pulse with profuse blood is the result of internal heat from drinking [alcohol]. (6) A large pulse with scant blood is the result of wind qì in the vessels but no intake of fluids. (7) This is what I mean."

I.10 Elaborating on Pricking by Section[*]
Cháng cì jié lùn
長刺節論

Note:

* Excerpted from *Sù Wèn* 55, *Cháng cì jié lùn* 長刺節論 (Elaborating on Pricking by Section).

Line 1

岐伯曰：刺家不診，聽病者言 。

Qíbó said: "The master of pricking[*] does not diagnose but [merely] listens to the patient's words.

Note:

* I.e., a skilled acupuncturist.

Line 2

(一)在頭，頭疾痛，為藏*針之，刺至骨病已 。(二)上無傷骨肉及皮 。(三)皮者道也 。

(1) If [the disease] is located in the head, with racing pain in the head, apply the needles there. Prick until you reach the bone and the disease is cured. (2) In the upper body, do not damage the bones, flesh, and skin. (3) The skin is the pathway [through which the needles enter the body].

Note:

    * I follow the commentary tradition according to which the character *zàng* 臟 (viscus) is a later addition to the text that should be deleted. Alternatively, the character is interpreted as *shén* 深 "deeply," so that the whole phrase means "insert the needles deeply."

Line 3

(一)陰¹刺，入一旁四處 。(二)治寒熱 。(三)深專者，刺大臟 。迫臟刺背，背俞也 。(四)刺之迫臟，臟會 。(五)腹中寒熱去而止 。(六)刺俞之要，發針而淺出血 。

(1) In [the technique of] yáng needling, insert one [needle straight in the center] and one each on the four sides. (2) [Use it] to treat [aversion to] cold and heat [effusion]. (3) If [the evil] has spread into the depth [of the body],² prick the major viscera.³ If [the evil] has come near the viscera, prick the back. This refers to the back transport points. (4) The place to prick [when evil] has come near the viscera is the meeting place of the viscera.⁴ (5) Stop when the cold and heat in the abdomen have been removed. (6) The important thing when pricking the transport points is to lift the needle up and superficially draw blood.

Notes:

    1. According to several parallel phrases in *Líng Shū*, *Zhēn Jiǔ Jiǎ Yǐ Jīng* 針灸甲乙經 (*A-Z Classic of Acupuncture and Moxibustion*), and *Tài Sù*, modern translators of *Sù Wèn* 55 interpret *yīn* 陰 here as a mistake that should be replaced with *yáng* 陽. *Líng Shū* 7, *guān zhēn* 官針 (Managing Needles) defines the yáng needling technique as applying one needle directly in the center and one needle on each of the four sides, as a treatment for heat and cold evil in the yáng aspect.
    2. I.e., into the yīn aspect of the body.
    3. According to most commentators, this refers to the alarm points of the five viscera, i.e. Zhōng Fǔ 中府 (LU-1) (lung), Zhāng Mén 章門 (LV-13) (spleen), Qī Mén 期門 (LV-14) (liver), Jīng Mén 京門 (GB-25) (kidney), and Jù Què 巨闕 (CV-14) (heart).
    4. There are two different commentary traditions on the meaning of the term *zàng huì* 臟會 ("meeting point of the viscera") here. According to one, this refers to the alarm points of all the five viscera (see previous note). According to the second, this is an alternative name specifically for Zhāng Mén, the point associated with the spleen.

Line 4

(一)治腐*腫者，刺腐上 。(二)視癰小大淺深刺 。(三)刺大者多血；小者深之 。(四)必端內針為故止 。

(1) To treat swollen welling-abscess, prick on top of the abscess. (2) Determine the depth of pricking by the size of the welling-abscess. (3) When pricking a large abscess, draw a lot of blood. For a small one, prick deeply. (4) You must insert the needle straight and then stop.

Note:

> * According to modern editions of the *Sù Wèn*, the character *fǔ* 腐 (putrify) should be replaced with *yōng* 癰 (welling-abscess), based on similar phrases in the *Zhēn Jiǔ Jiǎ Yǐ Jing* and *Tài Sù*.

Line 5

(一)病在少腹有積，刺皮䯏以下，至少腹而止 。(二)刺俠脊兩旁四椎間，刺兩髂髎季脅肋間 。(三)導腹中氣熱下已 。

(1) If disease is located in the lesser abdomen [with the key symptom being] accumulations, prick below the thick skin and stop when you reach the lesser abdomen. (2) Also prick on both sides of the spine at the fourth vertebra, as well as on both sides of the pelvis at the Jū Liáo (GB-29) points and at Jì Xié (LV-13) between the ribs. (3) Guide the hot qì in the abdomen downward, and the patient will recover.

Line 6

(一)病在少腹，腹痛、不得大小便，病名曰疝 。(二)得之寒 。(三)刺少腹兩股間，刺腰髁骨間，刺而多之，盡炅病已 。

(1) If the disease is located in the lesser abdomen [with the key symptoms being] abdominal pain and inability to urinate or defecate, the disease is called mounting. (2) It is the result of contracting cold. (3) Prick the lesser abdomen and both thighs, as well as between the lumbus and hip. Prick many [points] there until the intense heat is all drawn out, and the disease is cured.

Line 7

(一)病在筋，筋攣節痛不可以行，名曰筋痹 。(二)刺筋上為故，刺分肉間，不可中骨也 。(三)病起筋炅，病已乃止 。

(1) If the disease is located in the sinews [with the key symptoms being] hypertonicity in the sinews and joint pain with inability to walk, this is called sinew impediment. (2) Prick on top of the sinews as your guiding principle. Prick between the seams of the flesh and do not hit the bones. (3) As the disease rises, the sinews become hot. [This means that] the disease is cured, so you can stop then.

Line 8

(一)病在肌膚，肌膚盡痛，名曰肌痹 。(二)傷於寒濕 。(三)刺大分 、小分，多發針而深之 。(四)以熱為故 。(五)無傷筋骨，傷筋骨癰發 。(六)若變諸分盡熱，病已止 。

(1) If disease is located in the flesh and skin [with the key symptom being] pain all over the flesh and skin, it is called flesh impediment. (2) It is caused by damage from cold-damp. (3) Prick the large seams and small seams,* raise the needle numerous times and insert it deeply. (4) Take heat as your guide. (5) Do not damage the sinews or bones. If you damage sinews or bones, a welling-abscess will arise. (6) If you cause change in the various seams and they all become hot, [this means that] the disease is cured and you may stop [the treatment].

Note:

    * According to modern commentary, this is supposed to refer to points where the large and small muscles meet.

Line 9

(一)病在骨，骨重不可舉 、骨髓痠痛 、寒氣至 、名曰骨痹 。(二)深者刺，無傷脈肉為故，其道大分 、小分，骨熱病已止 。

(1) If the disease is located in the bones with [the key symptoms being] heaviness in the bones so that the patient cannot lift them, soreness and pain in the bones and

marrow, and cold qì arriving [in the bones], this is called bone impediment. (2) Prick deeply but do not damage the vessels and flesh, taking this as your guiding principle. The pathway [of the needle] should be in the large seams and small seams. Heat in the bones means that the disease is cured, and you may stop [the treatment].

Line 10

（一）病在諸陽脈，且寒且熱，諸分且寒且熱曰狂 。（二）刺之虛脈，視分盡熱病已止 。

(1) If the disease is in the various yáng vessels with [the key symptom being] both [aversion to] cold and heat [effusion], and the various seams also showing both [aversion to] cold and heat [effusion], it is called mania. (2) Prick [the yáng vessels] to make them vacuous.* When you see that the seams are hot all over, the disease is cured and you may stop [the treatment].

Note:

    * I.e., use a draining technique to dissipate the evil qì from the affected vessel.

Line 11

（一）病初發，歲一發；不治，月一發；不治，月四五發 。（二）名曰癲病 。（三）刺諸分諸脈 。（四）其無寒者，以針調之，病已止 。

(1) There is a disease that when it first arises, erupts once a year. If left untreated, it erupts once a month. If left untreated, it erupts four or five times a month. (2) This disease is called withdrawal disease.* (3) Prick the various seams and the various vessels. (4) If there are no cold symptoms, you can use needles to regulate it. Stop when the disease is cured.

Note:

    * *Diān* 癲 is now often associated with the biomedical condition of epilepsy.

Line 12

(一)病風且寒熱，炅汗出，一日數過 。(二)先刺諸分理脈絡 。(三)汗出，且寒且熱，三日一刺，百日而已 。

(1) Wind disease is characterized by both [aversion to] cold and heat [effusion], and by intense heat with sweating that occurs several times a day. (2) First prick the various seams, interstices, vessels, and network vessels. (3) When there is sweating with both [aversion to] cold and heat [effusion], prick once every three days. After a hundred days, the patient will have recovered.

Line 13

(一)病大風，骨節重 、鬚眉墮 、名曰大風 。(二)刺肌肉為故，汗出百日 。(三)刺骨髓，汗出百日，凡二百日 。(四)鬚眉生而止針 。

(1) If a patient suffers from great wind, [the key symptoms are] heaviness in the bones and joints and hair loss in the beard and eyebrows. This is called great wind. (2) Take pricking the flesh as your guiding principle and make the patient sweat for 100 days. (3) Then, prick the bone and marrow and make the patient sweat for another 100 days, for a total treatment length of 200 days. (4) When the beard and eyebrows grow back, stop needling."

I.11 On the Region of the Skin*
Pí bù lùn
皮部論

Note:

    * Excerpted from *Sù Wèn* 56, *Pí bù lùn* 皮部論 (On the Region of the Skin).

Line 1

帝曰：皮之十二部，其生病皆何如？

The [Yellow] Emperor said: "The skin has twelve regions. How do each of these generate disease?"

Line 2

(一)岐伯曰：皮者，脈之部也 。(二)邪客於皮，則腠理開 。開則邪入，客於絡脈 。絡脈滿則注於經脈 。經脈滿，則入舍於腑臟也 。(三)故皮者有分部，不與*而生大病也 。

(1) Qíbó said: "The skin is [divided into] sections associated with the vessels. (2) When evil lodges in the skin, the interstices open. As they open, the evil enters and lodges in the network vessels. As the network vessels become full, [their contents] pour into the channels. As the channels become full, [the evil] enters to take up residence in the viscera and bowels. (3) For this reason, the skin is divided into sections. If it is not healed, it will generate major illness."

Note:

    * According to some commentators on *Sù Wèn* 55 and the present text, and on the basis of a similar phrase in the *Zhēn Jiǔ Jiǎ Yǐ Jīng*, *yǔ* 與 should be replaced with *yù* 愈 ("heal"). I have translated accordingly.

I.12 On the Channels and Network Vessels*
Jīng luò lùn
經絡論

Note:

> * Excerpted from *Sù Wèn* 57, *Jīng luò lùn* 經絡論 (On the Channels and Network Vessels).

Line 1

(一)黃帝問曰：夫絡脈之見也，其五色各異，青、黃、赤、白、黑不同，其故何也？(二)岐伯對曰：經有常色，而絡無常變也。

(1) The Yellow Emperor asked: "Now as for the appearance of the network vessels, they each manifest differently in the five colors, in green-blue, yellow, red, white, and black. What is the reason for that?" (2) Qíbó answered: "The channels have their constant colors, but the network vessels do not have their constant color but change."

Line 2

(一)帝曰：經之常色何如？(二)曰：心赤、肺白、肝青、脾黃、腎黑、皆亦應其經脈之色也。

(1) The Emperor asked: "What are the constant colors of the channels?" (2) Qíbó replied: "The heart is red, the lung white, the liver green-blue, the spleen yellow, and the kidney black. All of these also correspond to the colors of the channels."

Line 3

(一)帝曰：絡之陰陽，亦應其經乎！(二)曰：陰絡之色應其經，陽絡之色變無常，隨四時而行也 。

(1) The Emperor said: "Alas, the yīn and yáng network vessels should also correspond to their channels!" (2) Qíbó replied: "The color of the yīn network vessels corresponds to their channels, but the color of the yáng network vessels changes without constancy, moving with the four seasons.

Line 4

(一)寒多則凝泣，凝泣則青黑 。(二)熱多則淖澤，淖澤則黃赤 。(三)此皆常色，謂之無病；五色具見者，謂之寒熱 。

(1) When there is a lot of cold, [the flow in the vessels] congeals and becomes blocked. As it congeals and becomes blocked, the result is a green-blue and black coloration. (2) When there is a lot of heat, the flow becomes slushy and moistened. As it becomes slushy and moistened, the result is a yellow and red coloration. (3) All of these are their constant colors. They are referred to as non-pathologic. If the five colors all manifest simultaneously, this is what is called cold and heat."

I.13 On the Empty Spaces by the Bones[*]
Gǔ kōng lùn
骨空論

Note:

    [*] Excerpted from *Sù Wèn* 60, *Gǔ kōng lùn* 骨空論 (On the Empty Spaces by the Bones).

Line 1

黃帝問曰：余聞風者，百病之始也 。以針治之奈何？

The Yellow Emperor asked: "I have heard that wind is the beginning of all disease. How do you treat it with needles?"

Line 2

(一) 岐伯對曰：風從外入，令人振寒 、汗出 、頭痛 、身重 、傷寒 。(二) 治在風府，調其陰陽 。(三) 不足則補，有餘則瀉 。

(1) Qíbó answered: "Wind enters the body from the outside and causes the person to suffer from quivering with cold, sweating, headache, generalized heaviness, and cold damage.[*] (2) Treat at Fēng Fǔ (GV-16) to regulate yīn and yáng. (3) In patients with insufficiency [of right qì], supplement. In patients with excess [of evil qì], drain.

Note:

    [*] *Sù Wèn* 60 has *wù hán* 惡寒 (aversion to cold) here instead of *shāng hán* 傷寒 (cold damage).

Line 3

（一）大風頸項痛，刺風府 。（二）大風汗出，灸譩譆，以手壓之，令病者呼譩譆，譩譆應手 。（三）從風憎風刺眉頭 。（四）失枕在肩上橫骨間，折使揄臂，齊肘，正灸脊中 。

(1) For great wind with pain in the nape and neck, prick Fēng Fǔ (GV-16). (2) For great wind with sweating, burn moxa at Yī Xǐ (BL-45). Use your hand and push down, making the patient call out 'Yixi!' Yī Xǐ responds to your hand.[1] (3) For patients who detest wind when facing it, prick Méi Tóu (BL-2).[2] (4) For a crick in the neck between the horizontal bones above the shoulders, have the patient bend the arms in such a way that the elbows are aligned and then apply moxa right in the middle of the spine.

Notes:

1. These latter two sentences explain how to identify the exact location of the point, below the sixth vertebra 3 *cùn* to each side of the spine. Because it is sensitive to pain, you press down in the area with a finger until the patient cries out in pain – and that is the point!

2. According to modern commentary, *méi tóu* 眉頭 is an alternate name for Zǎn Zhú 攢竹 (BL-2).

Line 4

（一）胅絡[1]季脅引少腹而痛脹，刺譩譆 。（二）腰痛不可以轉搖，急引陰卵，刺八髎與痛上 。（三）八髎在腰尻分間 。

(1) For pain and distention stretching from Jì Xié (LV-13) below the rib-sides to the lesser abdomen, prick Yī Xǐ (BL-45). (2) For lumbar pain with inability to turn sides or move, and tension stretching to the testicles, prick the Bā Liáo points[2] and on top of the place where it is painful. (3) The Bā Liáo points are found between the lumbus and the coccyx.

Notes:

1. *Miǎo luò* is the name of a network vessel located in the soft hollow area below the rib-sides.
2. This refers to the two Shàng Liáo 上髎 (BL-31), Cì Liáo 次髎 (BL-32), Zhōng Liáo 中髎 (BL-33), and Xià Liáo 下髎 (BL-34) points on both sides of the spine.

Line 5

（一）鼠瘰寒熱還，刺寒府 。（二）寒府在附膝外解營 。（三）取膝上外者，使之拜，取足心者，使之跪也 。

(1) For mouse fistula with recurrent [aversion to] cold and heat [effusion], prick Hán Fǔ (GB-33). (2) Hán Fǔ is located in the space between the joints on the outside of the knee. (3) To find the points on the outside on top of the knee, make the patient bend as if praying.* To find the points on the sole of the feet, make the patient kneel."

Note:

* I.e., keep the lower body straight and only bend the upper body.

I.14 On Pricking Water and Heat Points*
Cì shuǐ rè xué lùn
刺水熱穴論

Note:

> * Excerpted from *Sù Wèn* 61, *Shuǐ rè xué lùn* 水熱穴論 (On Pricking Water and Heat Points).

Line 1

黃帝問曰：少陰何以主腎，腎何以主水？

The Yellow Emperor asked: "How is it that the shàoyīn [vessel] governs the kidney and that the kidney governs water?"

Line 2

(一)岐伯曰：腎者，至陰也。(二)至陰者，盛水也。(三)肺者，太陰也。
(四)少陰者，冬脈也。(五)故其本在腎，其末在肺，皆積水也。

(1) Qíbó said: "The kidney is consummate yīn. (2) Consummate yīn is exuberant water. (3) The lung is tàiyīn.* (4) Shàoyīn is the vessel of winter. (5) For this reason, its root is in the kidney and its tip in the lung. Both of these accumulate water."

Note:

> * Literally, the terms "tàiyīn" and "shàoyīn" mean "greater yīn" and "lesser yīn."

Line 3

帝曰：腎何以能聚水而生病？

The Emperor asked: "How is it that the kidney is able to gather water and engender disease?"

Line 4

(一)岐伯曰：腎者，胃之關也 。(二)關門不利，故聚水，而從其類也 。
(三)上下溢於皮膚，故為胕腫 。(四)胕腫者，聚水而生病也 。

(1) Qíbó said: "The kidney is the barrier to the stomach. (2) If the gate in the barrier is inhibited, it causes water to gather, and diseases of this category follow. (3) Because [water] spills into the skin above and below [the kidney], it causes puffy swelling. (4) Puffy swelling is a disease caused by gathering water."

Line 5

帝曰：諸水皆生於腎乎？

The Emperor said: "Do all water [disorders] start in the kidney?"

Line 6

(一)曰：腎者牝臟也 。(二)地氣上者屬於腎，而生水液也，故曰至陰 。(三)勇而勞甚，則腎汗出 。(四)腎汗出逢於風，內不得入於臟腑，外不得越於皮膚，客於玄府，行於皮裏，傳為胕腫 。(五)本之於腎，名曰風水，所謂玄府者，汗孔也 。

(1) [Qíbó] said: "The kidney is the female viscus.* (2) The rise of earth qì is associated with the kidney, and it engenders the fluids. Therefore it is called consummate yīn. (3) Courage that results in great taxation makes the kidney sweat. (4) When the person encounters wind while the kidney is sweating, [the sweat] is unable to enter the viscera and bowels on the inside of the body or to float astray through the skin on the outside, but lodges in the mysterious mansions and moves into the skin where it transforms into puffy swelling. (5) The root of this condition is in the kidney and it is

called 'wind water.' What I mean by the mysterious mansions is the sweat pores."

Note:

* In this context meaning that it is the viscus most strongly associated with yīn.

Line 7

帝曰：水俞五十七處者，是何主也？

The Emperor said: "The 57 locations of the water transport points,* how are they governed?"

Note:

* I.e., the points used in acumoxa therapy for treating water-related disorders.

Line 8

(一)岐伯曰：腎俞五十七穴，積陰之所聚也，水所從出入也。(二)尻上五行，行五者，此腎俞。(三)故水病下為胕腫大腹，上為喘呼，不得臥者。(四)標本俱病，故肺為喘呼，腎為水腫，肺為逆不得臥，分為相輸，俱受者，水氣之所留也。(五)伏兔上各二行，行五者，此腎之街也。(六)三陰之所交結於腳也。(七)踝上各一行，行六者，此腎脈之下行也。名曰太衝。(八)凡五十七穴者，皆臟之陰絡，水之所客也。

(1) Qíbó said: "The 57 kidney transport points are where accumulations of yīn gather and where water exits and enters. (2) On top of the coccyx, there are five lines, and on the five lines, this is where the kidney transport points are located. (3) Thus, water disease manifests in puffy swelling and an enlarged abdomen in the lower body and in panting and sleeplessness in the upper body. (4) The root and tip are both diseased, as a result of which the lung manifests with panting, and the kidney with water swelling, and [we see] counterflow and sleeplessness in the lung. They manifest differently but affect each other. The reason why they both have contracted disease is that water qì has lodged there. (5) Above Fú Tù (ST-32), there are two lines on each side with five points on each of them. These are the thoroughfares of the kidney.

87

(6) The foot is where the three yīn [channels][1] intersect. (7) On top of the ankle, there is one line each with six points on each of them. These are where the kidney vessel runs downward. They are called Tài Chōng. (8) All of these 57 points are on the yīn network vessels of the viscera[2] and in places where water has settled."

Notes:

1. I.e. the kidney, liver, and spleen channels.
2. In one edition of *Sù Wèn* 61, the character *zàng* 臟 (viscus) is written without the radical as *cáng* 藏 and interpreted as "hidden deeply inside the body." The interchangeable use of related characters is a common problem with early texts because characters were so often written without the correct radical and the interpretation left to the reader on the basis of the specific context.

Line 9

帝曰：春取絡脈分肉何也？

The Emperor said: "Why is that in the spring we select the network vessels at the seam of the flesh [to treat patients with acupuncture]?"

Line 10

曰：春者，木始治，肝氣如生，肝氣急，其風疾，經脈常深，其氣少，不能深入，故取絡脈分肉間 。

Qíbó said: "In the spring, wood begins to rule and liver qì likewise is engendered. Liver qì is urgent and its wind is racing. The channel[1] is normally deep and its qì[2] is scant. Unable to enter deeply, we therefore select the network vessels at the seam of the flesh."

Notes:

1. This could refer to the liver channel specifically, or the channels in general, in contrast to the network vessels. It also has the connotation of the pulse in the vessel.
2. Again, this could refer to the person's qì in general (or specifically their yáng qì), to their liver qì more specifically, or to wind qì.

Line 11

帝曰：夏取盛經分腠何也？

The Emperor said: "Why is it that in the summer we select the exuberant channels at the seam of the interstices?"

Line 12

（一）曰：夏者，火始治，心氣始長，脈瘦氣弱，陽氣流溢，熱熏分腠，內至於經，故取盛經分腠。（二）絕膚而病去者，邪居淺也。（三）所謂盛經者，陽脈也。

(1) [Qíbó] said: "In the summer, fire begins to rule and heart qì begins to grow. The vessels are emaciated and the qì is weak, but the flow of yáng qì spills forth. Heat fumes in the seams of the interstices and reaches the channels on the inside. Therefore we select the exuberant channels at the seam of the interstices. (2) The reason that we merely pierce through the skin and make the disease leave is because the evil resides in the shallow [layer of the body]. (3) What I mean by exuberant channels is the yáng vessels."

Line 13

帝曰：秋取經俞何也？

The Emperor said: "Why is it that in the fall we select the transport points on the channels?"

Line 14

（一）曰：秋者，金始治，肺將收殺，金將勝火，陽氣在合，陰氣初勝。（二）濕氣及體，陰氣未盛，未能深入，故取俞以瀉陰邪，取合以虛陽邪，陽氣始衰故取於合。

(1) [Qíbó] said: "In the fall, metal begins to rule and the lung receives and kills. Metal is about to overcome fire. Yáng qì is located at the uniting points, and yīn qì begins to overcome. (2) When damp qì reaches the body, yīn qì is not yet exuberant and it

is unable to enter deeply. Hence we select the transport points to drain yīn evil and we select the uniting points to empty yáng evil. Because yáng qì begins to weaken, we select the uniting points."

Line 15

帝曰：冬取井榮何也？

The Emperor said: "Why is it that in the winter we select the well and brook points?"

Line 16

（一）曰：冬者，水始治，腎方閉，陽氣衰少，陰氣堅盛，巨陽伏沉，陽氣乃去。（二）故取井以下陰逆，取榮以實陽氣。（三）故曰冬取井榮，春不鼽衄，此之謂也。

(1) [Qíbó] said: "In the winter, water begins to govern and the kidney is closing up. Yáng qì is debilitated and scant, and yīn qì is firm and exuberant. The tàiyáng [vessel] is hidden deeply and yáng qì follows it there. (2) Hence we select the well points to precipitate counterflow yīn qì and we select the brook points to make yáng qì replete. (3) Therefore I say: 'If you select the well and brook points in the winter, there will be no nasal congestion and nosebleed in the spring.' This is what I mean by that."

Line 17

帝曰：夫子言，治熱病五十九俞。願聞其處，因聞其義。

The Emperor said: "Master, you have already discussed using the 59 transport points for treating heat disease. I would now like to hear about their location and then about their significance."

Line 18

(一)岐伯曰：頭上五行，行五者，以越諸陽之熱逆也 。(二)大杼 、膺俞 、缺盆 、背俞 、此八者，以瀉胸中之熱也 。(三)氣街 、三里 、巨虛上下廉，此八者，以瀉胃中之熱也 。(四)雲門 、髃骨 、委中 、髓空，此八者以瀉四肢之熱也 。(五)五臟俞旁五，此十者，以瀉五臟之熱也 。(六)凡此五十九穴者，皆熱之左右也 。

(1) **Qíbó said:** "There are five lines on top of the head with five points on each line. They are used to lead astray the heat counterflow in the various yáng [vessels]. (2) Dà Zhù (BL-11), Yīng Shū (LU-1), Quē Pén (ST-12), and Bèi Shù,[1] these eight points are used to drain heat from inside the chest. (3) Qì Jiē (ST-30), Sān Lǐ (ST-36), and upper and lower Jù Xū (ST-37 and -39 respectively), these eight points are used to drain heat from inside the stomach. (4) Yún Mén (LU-2), Yú Gǔ (LI-15),[2] Wěi Zhōng (BL-40), and Suí Kǒng (GV-2), these eight points are used to drain heat from the four limbs. (5) The five points besides the transport points for the five viscera, these ten points are used to drain heat from the five viscera. (6) Altogether these 59 points are to the left or right of heat."[3]

Notes:

1. Bèi Shù 背俞 (lit. "back transport point") can be interpreted as either BL-15 or BL-11.
2. This point is identical with the modern point Jiān Yú 肩髃 (LI-15).
3. Depending on interpretation, this somewhat obscure line could mean that these points all treat heat, whether [the points OR the heat] are located on the left or right, or it could mean that they are located in the general vicinity of the heat.

Line 19

帝曰：人傷於寒，而傳為熱，何也？

The Emperor said: "How is it that when a person is damaged by cold, it can transform into heat?"

Line 20

岐伯曰：夫寒盛，則生熱也 。

Qíbó said: "When cold is exuberant, it engenders heat."

I.15 On Regulating the Channels[*]
Tiáo jīng lùn
調經論

Notes:

    [*] Excerpted from *Sù Wèn* 62, *Tiáo jīng lùn* 調經論 (On Regulating the Channels).

Line 1

黃帝問曰：有餘不足 。余已聞虛實之形，不知何以生？

The Yellow Emperor asked: "There are [conditions of] excess and there are [conditions of] insufficiency. I have already heard about the form of vacuity and repletion,[*] but I do not know how they are engendered."

Note:

    [*] This is a reference to the preceding paragraphs in *Sù Wèn* 62, which discuss the manifestations and treatment of excess and vacuity in the spirit (*shén* 神) qì (*qì* 氣), blood (*xuè* 血), physical body (*xíng* 形), and will (*zhì* 志).

Line 2

(一)岐伯曰：氣血已并，陰陽相傾，氣亂於衛，血逆於經，血氣離居一實一虛。(二)血并於陰，氣并於陽，故為驚狂。血并於陽，氣并於陰，乃為炅中。血并於上。(三)氣并於下，心煩惋喜怒。血并於下，氣并於上，亂而喜忘。

(1) **Qíbó said: "Qì and blood combine [in abnormal concentrations],[1] yīn and yáng are out of balance with each other, qì is chaotic in the defense, blood runs counterflow in the channels, and qì and blood reside separate from each other, one replete and the other vacuous. (2) When blood combines in yīn and qì combines in yáng, this causes fright and mania. When blood combines in yáng and qì combines in yīn, this causes intense heat in the center. (3) When blood combines above[2] and qì combines below, we see vexation in the heart, sighing, and irascibility. When blood combines below and qì combines above, we see chaos and forgetfulness."**

Notes:

1. In this context, *bìng* 並 does not mean that qì and blood combine WITH EACH OTHER, but rather that each of them gathers in abnormal concentrations in different aspects of the body. While "concentrate" may be a more elegant translation here, I have chosen to retain the more literal meaning of "combine" because that is what the Chinese character says.
2. According to some commentators, above and below refer to above and below the diaphragm. More commonly, though, the terms *shàng* 上 and *xià* 下 refer to the upper and lower half of the body.

Line 3

帝曰：血并於陰，氣并於陽，如是血氣離居，何者為實？ 何者為虛？

The Emperor said: "When blood combines in yīn while qì combines in yáng, so that blood and qì reside separate from each other in this way, which one is replete? Which one is vacuous?"

Line 4

(一)岐伯曰：血氣者喜溫而惡寒，寒則泣不能流，溫則消而去之 。(二)是故氣之所并為血虛，血之所并為氣虛 。

(1) Qíbó said: "Qì and blood have a liking for warmth and an aversion to cold. When they are cold, they become blocked and unable to flow; when they are warm, they are dispersed and leave from there. (2) For this reason, blood is vacuous where qì is combined and qì is vacuous where blood is combined."

Line 5

(一)帝曰：人之所有者，血與氣爾 。(二)今夫子乃言，血并為虛，氣并為虛，是無實乎！

(1) The Emperor said: "Humans have both blood and qì. (2) Now what you, Master, are saying is that the combining of blood causes vacuity [of qì] and that the combining of qì causes vacuity [of blood]. But in this way, there is no repletion!"

Line 6

(一)岐伯曰：有者為實，無者為虛，故氣并則無血，血并則無氣 。(二)今血與氣相失，故為虛焉 。(三)絡之與孫脈，俱輸於經，血與氣並，則為實焉 。(四)血之與氣，并走於上，則為大厥，厥則暴死 。(五)氣復反則生，不反則死 。

(1) Qíbó said: "When something is present, it means repletion. When something is absent, it means vacuity. Therefore, the combining of qì results in an absence of blood, and the combining of blood results in an absence of qì. (2) In the present situation, blood and qì have lost each other, hence this means vacuity there. (3) The network vessels and ancestral vessels all transport [blood and qì] back to the channels. When blood and qì combine, this means repletion there. (4) When blood and qì in combination run into the upper body, the result is major reversal. When there is reversal, sudden death results. (5) When qì again reverses direction [and returns to the lower body], life results. When it fails to reverse direction, death results."

Line 7

帝曰：實者何道從來，虛者何道從去，虛實之要，願聞其故 。

The Emperor said: "Which path does repletion come from? Which path does vacuity leave on? I would like to hear the rationale for the principles of vacuity and repletion."

Line 8

(一)岐伯曰：夫陰與陽，皆有俞會，陽注於陰，陰滿之外 。(二)陰陽匀平，以充其形，九候若一，命曰平人 。(三)夫邪之生也，或生於陽，或生於陰 。(四)其生於陽者，得之風雨寒暑；其生於陰者，得之飲食居處，陰陽喜怒 。

(1) Qíbó said: "Now, the yīn and yáng [vessels] all have transport points where they meet. Yáng pours into yīn and yīn fills what flows to the outside. (2) Yīn and yáng thus establish a mutual balance and thereby fill the physical body. The nine indicators [of pulse diagnosis] appear as one. This is what is called a balanced person. (3) Now as for evil being engendered, it can either be engendered in yáng or it can be engendered in yīn. (4) When engendered in yáng, it is contracted from wind, rain, cold, or summerheat; when engendered in yīn, it is contracted from [inappropriate] food and drink and dwellings, sexual intercourse, and irascibility."

Line 9

帝曰：風雨之傷人奈何？

The Emperor said: "How is it that wind and rain damage a person?"

Line 10

(一)曰：風雨之傷人也，先客於皮膚，傳入於孫脈。(二)孫脈滿則傳入於絡脈，絡脈滿則輸於大經脈。(三)血氣與邪並客於分腠之間。(四)其脈堅大，故曰實。(五)實者外堅充滿，不可按之，按之則痛。

(1) [Qíbó] said: "Here is the way in which wind and rain damage a person: They first settle in the skin and then spread to the ancestral vessels. (2) When the ancestral vessels are full, they spread to the network vessels. When the network vessels are full, they move to the major channels. (3) Qì and blood combine with the evil and settle in the seams and intestices. (4) The person's vessels become firm and enlarged. Hence we speak of repletion. (5) Repletion refers to the outside being firm and full so that you are unable to press down on it. If you do press down, pain results."

Line 11

帝曰：寒濕之傷人奈何？

The Emperor said: "How is it that cold and dampness damage a person?"

Line 12

(一)曰：寒濕之中人也，皮膚不收，肌肉堅緊，榮血泣，衛氣去。故曰虛。(二)虛者聶辟，氣不足，按之則氣足以溫之，故快然而不痛。

(1) [Qíbó] said: "Here is the way in which cold and dampness strike a person: The skin fails to contract, the flesh is firm and tight, construction blood is congealed and defense qì has left. Hence we speak of vacuity. (2) Vacuity [disease is characterized by] wrinkles in the skin with insufficiency of qì. If you push down on [the place where the vacuity is located], qì becomes sufficient and the patient feels warmth there. Therefore the patient is happy and free of pain."

Line 13

帝曰：陰之生實奈何？

The Emperor said: "How is it that yīn engenders repletion?"

96

Line 14

曰：喜怒不節，則陰氣上逆，上逆則下虛，下虛則陽氣走之，故曰實矣 。

[Qíbó] said: "Irascibility without moderation results in counterflow ascent of yīn qì. This counterflow ascent results in vacuity below. Vacuity below causes yáng qì to go there. Hence we speak of repletion."

Line 15

帝曰：陰之生虛奈何？

The Emperor said: "How is it that yīn engenders vacuity?"

Line 16

曰：喜則氣下，悲則氣消，消則脈虛空，因寒飲食，寒氣熏滿，則血泣氣去，故曰虛矣 。

[Qíbó] said: "Joy causes qì to descend. Grief causes qì to disperse. When qì disperses, the vessels are empty. Due to cold drink and food, cold qì fumes and causes fullness. As a result, blood congeals and qì leaves. Therefore we speak of vacuity."

Line 17

(一)帝曰：經言陽虛則外寒 ； 陰虛則內熱 ； 陽盛則外熱 ； 陰盛則內寒 。
(二)余已聞之矣，不知其所由然也 。

(1) The Emperor said: "As the classics say, 'yáng vacuity results in cold on the outside; yīn vacuity results in heat on the inside; yáng exuberance results in heat on the outside; yīn exuberance results in cold on the inside.' (2) I would like to hear [more] about this. I do not know the reason why this is so."

Line 18

(一)岐伯曰：陽受氣於上焦，以溫皮膚分肉之間 。(二)今寒氣在外，則上焦不通，上焦不通，則寒氣獨於外，故寒慄 。

(1) Qíbó said: "Yáng receives qì in the upper burner* and thereby warms the space between skin and the seam of the flesh. (2) Now when there is cold qì on the outside, stoppage in the upper burner results. When the upper burner is stopped up, cold qì remains only on the outside. Therefore we see [aversion to] cold and shivering."

Note:

* I.e., in the lung. As the result of exterior cold, the function of the lung to diffuse qì breaks down.

Line 19

帝曰：陰虛生內熱奈何？

The Emperor said: "How is it that yīn vacuity engenders heat on the inside?"

Line 20

曰：有所勞倦，形氣衰少，穀氣不盛，上焦不行，下脘不通，胃氣熱，熱氣薰胸中，故內熱 。

[Qíbó] said: "In cases of taxation fatigue, the qì of the physical body is weakened and scant,* grain qì is not exuberant, the upper burner fails to move [clear qì], and there is no flow through the lower stomach duct. Stomach qì becomes hot, and hot qì fumes [upward] into the chest. Hence internal heat results."

Note:

* This is a reference to the spleen, which has the function of absorbing the qì of food and drink.

Line 21

帝曰：陽盛生外熱奈何？

The Emperor said: "How is it that yáng exuberance engenders heat on the outside?"

Line 22

曰：上焦不通利，則皮膚緻密，腠理閉塞，玄府不通，衛氣不得泄越，故外熱。

[Qíbó] said: "When the upper burner is stopped up, the skin becomes tight, the interstices are obstructed, the sweat pores are stopped up, and defense qì is unable to discharge and effuse. Hence heat results on the outside."

Line 23

帝曰：陰盛生內寒奈何？

The Emperor said: "How is it that yīn exuberance engenders cold on the inside?"

Line 24

曰：厥氣上逆，寒氣積於胸中而不瀉，不瀉則溫氣去，寒獨留則血凝泣，凝則脈不通，其脈盛大以濇，故中寒。

[Qíbó] said: "Reversal qì ascends counterflow and cold qì gathers in the chest, failing to drain. If it does not drain, warm qì leaves and cold alone remains. As a result, blood congeals, and congealing results in stoppage in the vessels. The vessels become filled up and enlarged, and therefore rough. Hence we see cold strike."

Line 25

帝曰：陰於陽并，血氣以並，病形已成，刺之奈何？

The Emperor said: "When yīn has combined with yáng, and blood and qì have subsequently combined, and disease therefore has already formed in the body, how do you go about pricking it?"

Line 26

(一)曰：刺此者取之經隧，取血於榮，取氣於衛 。(二)用形哉，因四時多少高下 。

(1) [Qíbó] answered: "To prick this condition, address it in the channel passages. Address the blood in the construction [aspect of the body] and address the qì in the defense [aspect of the body]. (2) In using the physical body, follow the four seasons, the amount [of qì and blood], and the location above and below."

Line 27

(一)帝曰：夫子言虛實者有十，生於五臟，五臟五脈耳 。(二)夫十二經脈，皆生其病 。今夫子獨言五臟 。(三)夫十二經脈者，皆絡三百六十五節，節有病，必被經脈 。(四)經脈之病，皆有虛實，何以合之？

(1) The Emperor said: "Now you have spoken of ten types of vacuity and repletion, their engenderment in the five viscera, and [the association] of the five vessels with the five viscera. (2) However, the twelve channels all engender their own diseases. Now you have only spoken of the five viscera. (3) Moreover, the twelve channels all branch out into 365 sections, and if the sections have a disease, this invariably spreads to the channels. (4) The diseases of the channels all [fall into the category of] vacuity or repletion. How do you make all these consistent?"

Line 28

(一)岐伯曰：五臟者故得六腑與表裏 。(二)經絡支節，各生虛實 。(三)其病所居，隨而調之 。

(1) Qíbó said: "The five viscera thus stand in an exterior-interior relationship with the six bowels. (2) The channels and network vessels, branches and joints each can engender vacuity or repletion. (3) Start from where the disease is located, follow it, and regulate there.

Line 29

(一)病在脈，調之血 。(二)病在血，調之絡 。(三)病在氣，調之衛 。(四)病在肉，調之分肉 。(五)病在筋，調之筋，燔針劫刺其下及與急者 。(六)病在骨，調之骨，焠針藥熨 。

(1) When the disease is in the vessels, regulate it in the blood. (2) When the disease is in the blood, regulate it in the network vessels. (3) When the disease is in the qì, regulate it in the defense. (4) When the disease is in the flesh, regulate it in the seams of the flesh. (5) When the disease is in the sinews, regulate it in the sinews. Heat the needle until glowing and prick to force out what is underneath until [you achieve a sensation of] tension. (6) When the disease is in the bones, regulate it in the bones. Heat the needle until red* or apply hot medicinal compresses.

Notes:

* According to Zhāng Jièbīn, *cuì zhēn* 焠針 describes a needling technique where the needle is heated until glowing BEFORE it is inserted, while *fán zhēn* 燔針 refers to a technique where the needle is only heated AFTER it is inserted into the patient. While the latter merely "uses fire qì to disperse cold evil," the former actually "not only creates warmth but is the only way to deal with bound cold poison."

Line 30

(一)病不知所痛，兩蹻為上 。(二)身形有痛，九候莫病，則繆刺之 。(三)痛
在於左而右脈病者，巨刺之 。(四)必謹察其九候，針道備矣 。

(1) If you do not know exactly where the location of the pain is in a disease, needling
Yīn Qiāo (KI-6) and Yáng Qiāo (BL-62) is supreme. (2) When there is pain in the
physical body but the nine pulse indicators do not yet show any disease, then use
misleading pricking[1] to treat it. (3) When the pain is on the left but the right pulse
indicates disease, use grand pricking[2] to treat it. (4) Always cautiously examine the
patient's nine pulse indicators, and the path of the needle will be prepared.

Notes:

1. See the following chapter, which explains this technique in detail.
2. See chapter I.18 below, which explains this technique in detail.

I.16 On Misleading Pricking*
Miù cì lùn
繆刺論

Note:

> * Excerpted from *Sù Wèn* 63, *Miù cì lùn* 繆刺論 (On Misleading Pricking).

Line 1

黃帝問曰：余聞繆刺，未得其義，何為繆刺？

The Yellow Emperor asked: "I would like to hear about misleading pricking.* I do not yet grasp its meaning. What is 'misleading pricking'?"

Note:

> * The translation of *miù cì* 繆刺 is a difficult issue that has led to much debate from Wáng Bīng, the 8th century *Sù Wèn* commentator, to contemporary scholars in China and the West alike. While Nigel Wiseman, for example, advocates an interpretation of *miù* 繆 as "crosswise" and therefore translates it as "cross needling method," Paul U. Unschuld devotes an entire section in his book *Huang Di Nei Jing Su Wen* to the discussion of what he translates as "Misleading Piercing and Grand Piercing" (chapter 10.4, pp. 274-278). In this chapter, he makes a convincing case, based partly on Wáng Bīng's commentary, that we should indeed read *miù* 繆 in the sense of "misleading," in the sense of contrary to our expectations. The contents of this chapter support Unschuld's reading, presenting a needling method by which the patient is pricked at places distant from the location of the disease, contrary to our normal expectations. I have therefore chosen to follow Unschuld's translation.

Line 2

(一)岐伯對曰：夫邪客於皮毛，入舍於孫絡 。(二)留而不去，閉塞不通，不得入於經，流溢於大絡，而生奇病也 。(三)夫邪客大絡者，左注右 、右注左 、上下左右，與經相干，而布於四末 。(四)其氣無常處，不入於經俞，命曰繆刺 。

(1) Qíbó replied: "As evil intrudes through the skin and body hair, it enters to lodge in the grandchild network vessels.[1] (2) When it remains there instead of leaving, it causes congestion and stopped flow. Unable to enter the channels, it spills over into the major network vessels and generates strange diseases. (3) When evil intrudes into the major network vessels, it pours from the left into the right [side of the body] and from the right into the left, above, below, left, and right, interfering with the flow in the channels and spreading to the four branches.[2] (4) Its qì has no constant dwelling place and it does not enter the channel transport points. [The appropriate treatment method] is called 'misleading pricking.'"

Notes:

1. I.e., the minor vessels branching off the network vessels.
2. I.e., the four limbs.

Line 3

(一)帝曰：願聞繆刺 。(二)以左取右，以右取左奈何？ (三)其與巨刺何以別之？

(1) The Emperor said: "I would like to hear about misleading pricking. (2) Why is it that you choose the right [side of the body] for treating [evil] in the left and the left [side of the body] for treating [evil] in the right? (3) And how do you distinguish it from 'grand pricking'?"

Line 4

(一)曰：邪客於經，左盛則右病，右盛則左病，亦有移易者 。(二)左痛未已，而右脈先病，如此者，必巨刺之 。(三)必中其經，非絡脈也 。(四)故絡病者，具痛與經脈繆處，故命曰繆刺 。

(1) [Qíbó] said: "As evil intrudes into the channels, exuberance in the left results in disease in the right, exuberance in the right results in disease in the left. Moreover, there are also conditions that have a tendency to move around. (2) When the pain on the left has not yet stopped but the vessels on the right first [indicate] disease, in situations like this, you must [treat with the technique of] grand pricking. (3) You must hit the channels, and not the network vessels. (4) Now in disease of the network vessels, all the pain and the pulses in the channels [that indicate disease] are located in misleading places. Therefore, the [proper treatment] method is called 'misleading pricking.'"

Line 5

帝曰：願聞繆刺奈何，取之何如？

The Emperor said: "I would like to hear more about misleading pricking. How do you choose [the points to prick]?"

Line 6

(一)對曰：邪客於足少陰之絡，令人卒心痛、暴脹、胸脅支滿。(二)無積者，刺然骨之前出血，如食頃而已 。(三)不已，左取右，右取左 。(四)病新發者，取五日已 。

(1) [Qíbó] answered: "If the evil lodges in the network vessels of the foot shàoyīn [vessel], it causes the person to suffer from sudden heart pain, violent distention, and propping fullness in the chest and rib-sides. (2) If there is no accumulation, prick in front of the blazing bone,* drawing blood. After about the time it takes to eat a meal, the patient should recover. (3) If the patient fails to recover, for disease on the left select points on the right, for disease on the right select points on the left. (4) If the disease has developed only recently, the patient should recover after treatment for five days.

Note:

    * *Rán gǔ* 然骨: This can refer either to the navicular bone or specifically to the point *Rán Gǔ* 然骨 (KI-2).

Line 7

(一)邪客於手少陽之絡，令人喉痹舌卷、口乾心煩、臂外廉痛、手不及頭。(二)刺手小指次指爪甲上，去端如韭葉，各一痏。(三)壯者立已，老者有頃已。(四)左取右，右取左。(五)此新病數日已。

(1) If the evil lodges in the network vessels of the hand shàoyáng [vessel], it causes the person to suffer from throat impediment, a curled tongue, dry mouth, heart vexation, pain on the outside edge of the arms, and inability to raise the arms to the head. (2) Prick the nail of the ring finger, about the breadth of a leaf of Chinese chives down from the end of the nail,* once on each side. (3) Strong patients will recover immediately. Old patients will recover in a while. (4) For disease on the left, select points on the right; for disease on the right, select points on the left. (5) If this is a newly arisen disease, the patient will recover in a number of days.

Note:

    * This is identifiable as the modern point Guān Chōng 關衝 (TB-1).

Line 8

(一)邪客於足厥陰之絡，令人卒疝，暴痛。(二)刺足大指爪甲上與肉交者，各一痏。(三)男子立已，女子有頃已。(四)左取右，右取左。

(1) If the evil lodges in the network vessels of the foot juéyīn [vessel], it causes the person to suffer from sudden mounting with violent pain. (2) Prick above the toenail on the big toe, where it meets the flesh,* once on each side. (3) Male patients will immediately recover, female patients will recover in a while. (4) For disease on the left, select points on the right; for disease on the right, select points on the left.

Note:

    * This can be identified with the modern point Dà Dūn 大敦 (LV-1).

Line 9

(一)邪客於足太陽之絡，令人頭項肩痛。(二)刺足小指爪甲上與肉交者，各一痏，立已。(三)不已，刺外踝下三痏。(四)左取右，右取左。(五)如食頃已。

(1) If the evil lodges in the network vessels of the foot tàiyáng [vessel], it causes the person to suffer from pain in the head, nape, and shoulders. (2) Prick above the toenail of the little toe, where it meets the flesh,[1] once on each side, and immediate recovery will ensue. (3) If the patient fails to recover, prick below the outer ankle,[2] three times. (4) For disease on the left, select points on the right; for disease on the right, select points on the left. (5) The patient will recover in about the time it takes to eat a meal.

Notes:

    1. This is identifiable as Zhì Yīn 至陰 (BL-67).
    2. This is identifiable as Jīn Mén 金門 (BL-63).

Line 10

(一)邪客於手陽明之絡，令人氣滿、胸中喘息而支胠、胸中熱。(二)刺手大指次指爪甲上，去端如韭葉，各一痏。(三)左取右，右取左。(四)如食頃已。

(1) If the evil lodges in the network vessels of the hand yángmíng [vessel], it causes the person to suffer from fullness of qì, panting in the chest, propped flanks, and heat inside the chest. (2) Prick above the nail of the index finger, about the breadth of a leaf of Chinese chives down from the end of the nail,* once on each side. (3) For disease on the left, select points on the right; for disease on the right, select points on the left. (4) The patient will recover in about the time it takes to eat a meal.

Note:

    * This is identifiable as the modern point Shāng Yáng 商陽 (LI-1).

Line 11

(一)邪於臂掌之間，不可得屈，刺其踝後。(二)先以指按之，痛乃刺之。
(三)以月死生為數，月生一日一痏，二日二痏，十五日十五痏，十六日十四
痏。

(1) If the evil lodges between the upper arm and the palm of the hand, preventing the patient from bending the arm, prick behind the wrist. (2) First, push down with your finger. Wherever you find pain, prick right there. (3) Determine the number of pricking by the waxing and waning of the moon. On the first day of the new moon, one; on the second day, two; on the fifteenth day, fifteen; on the sixteenth day, fourteen.*

Note:

    * What is left out according to many scholars is that the number of recommended needle applications increases with the waxing moon and decreases with the waning moon. Hence you start decreasing the number once you have passed the fifteenth day, when the moon begins to wane. This is obviously premised on the notion that the qì in the human body corresponds to the qì in the universe, both of which are affected by or reflected in the qì of the moon. The state of the moon's qì is easily identified by glancing at the night sky: greatest during the full moon and weakest during the new moon.

Line 12

(一)邪客於足陽蹻之脈，令人目痛，從內眥始。(二)刺外踝之下半寸所，各
二痏。(三)左刺右，右刺左。(四)如行十里頃而已。

(1) If the evil lodges in the Yáng Qiāo vessel of the foot, it causes the person to suffer from eye pain, beginning from the inner canthus. (2) Prick the point that is located half a *cùn* below the outer ankle,[1] twice on each side. (3) For disease on the left, prick the right; for disease on the right, prick the left.[2] (4) The patient will recover in about the time it takes to walk ten *lǐ*.

Notes:

1. Identifiable as Shēn Mài 申脈 (BL-62).
2. I.e., select points on the right side of the body if the disease is located on the left side of the body and vice versa.

Line 13

(一)人有所墮墜，惡血留內，腹中滿脹、不得前後。(二)先飲利藥。(三)此上傷厥陰之脈，下傷少陰之絡。(四)刺足內踝之下，然骨之前，血脈出血。(五)刺足跗上動脈。(六)不已，刺三毛上，各一痏，見血立已。(七)左刺右，右刺左。(八)善悲驚不樂，刺如上方。

(1) If a person has had a falling accident, as a result of which malign blood is retained internally, [the key symptoms are] fullness and distention in the abdomen and inability to urinate or defecate. (2) First make the person drink disinhibiting medicine. (3) This patient has damaged the juéyīn vessel in the upper body and the network vessels of the shàoyīn [vessel] in the lower body. (4) Prick below the foot's inner ankle, in front of the blazing bone,[1] on the blood vessel,[2] drawing blood. (5) Also prick the stirring vessel on top of the dorsum.[3] (6) If the patient fails to recover, prick the width of three hairs above this point,[4] three times on each side. When you see blood, immediate recovery will ensue. (7) For disease on the left, prick the right; for disease on the right, prick the left. (8) If patients suffer from a tendency to grief, fright, and lack of joy, prick according to the above method.

Notes:

1. See the note above under line 6, same chapter
2. Some commentators identify this point as Zhōng Fēng 中封 (LV-4).
3. I.e., Chōng Yáng 衝陽 (ST-42).
4. Identified as Dà Dūn 大敦 (LV-1).

Line 14

(一)邪於手陽明之絡，令人耳聾，時不聞音。(二)刺手大指次指爪甲上，去
端如韭葉，各一痏，立聞。(三)不已，刺中指爪甲上與肉交者，立聞。(四)
其不時聞者，不可刺也。(五)耳中生風者，亦刺之如此數。(六)左刺右，右
刺左。

(1) If the evil is located in the network vessels of the hand yángmíng [vessel], it causes the patient to suffer from deafness that intermittently prevents the person from hearing sounds. (2) Prick on top of the nail of the index finger, about the breadth of a leaf of Chinese chives down from the end of the nail,[1] once on each side, and the patient's hearing will recover. (3) If no recovery ensues, prick above the nail of the middle finger where it meets the flesh,[2] and the patient's hearing will recover. (4) If the patient is unable to hear anything at any time at all, you cannot [treat it by] pricking.[3] (5) For wind engendered in the ears,[4] also prick in this fashion, repeatedly. (6) For disease on the left, prick the right; for disease on the right, prick the left.

Notes:

1. See the note above under line 10, same chapter. Identified as Shāng Yáng 商陽 (LI-1).
2. Identified as Zhōng Chōng 中衝 (PC-9).
3. The reason for this prohibition is that the condition is not caused by the presence of external evil in the body but by an internal condition that needs to be treated with different strategies.
4. Manifesting in tinnitus and the constant sound of blowing wind in the ears.

Line 15

(一)凡痺往來，行常處者，在分肉間痛而刺之。(二)以月死生為數。(三)用
針者，隨氣盛衰以為痏數。(四)針過其日數則脫氣，不及日數，則氣不瀉。
(五)左刺右，右刺左，病已止。(六)不已，復刺之如法。(七)月生一日一
痏，二日二痏，漸多之，十五日十五痏。(八)十六日十四痏，漸少之。

(1) For all cases of impediment that comes and goes and moves around in the body, [feel] where there is pain in the seams of the flesh and prick there. (2) Determine the number [of prickings] by the waxing and waning of the moon. (3) In using needles, you must follow the exuberance or debilitation of qì to determine the number of prickings. (4) If the needles exceed the number appropriate for that day, you will

cause qì desertion. If you do not reach the number appropriate for the day, the [evil] qì will not get drained. (5) For disease on the left, prick the right; for disease on the right, prick the left, and the disease will stop. (6) If it does not stop, again prick it by the above method. (7) On the first day of the waxing moon once, on the second day twice, gradually increasing the number to 15 times on the fifteenth day [of the waxing moon]. (8) On the sixteenth day, prick it fourteen times and then gradually decrease the number.

Line 16

(一) 邪客於足陽明之絡，令人鼻衄，上齒寒 。(二) 刺足大指次指爪甲上與肉交者，各一痏 。(三) 左刺右，右刺左 。

(1) If the evil lodges in the network vessels of the foot yángmíng [vessel], it causes the person to suffer from nosebleed and cold in the upper teeth. (2) Prick the toe next to the big toe above the nail where it meets the flesh,* once on each side. (3) For disease on the left, prick the right; for disease on the right, prick the left.

Note:

* Identified as Lì Duì 厲兌 (ST-45).

Line 17

(一) 邪客於足少陽之絡，令人脅痛 、不得息 、欬而汗出 。(二) 刺足小指次指爪甲上與肉交者，各一痏 。(三) 不得息立已；汗出立止；欬者，溫衣飲食，一日已 。(四) 左刺右，右刺左 。(五) 病立已 。不已，復刺如法 。

(1) If the evil lodges in the network vessels of the foot shàoyáng [vessel], it causes the person to suffer from pain in the rib-sides and inability to breathe, coughing, and sweating. (2) Prick the toe next to the little toe above the nail where it meets the flesh, once on each side.* (3) The inability to breathe will stop immediately, the sweating will stop immediately, and the coughing will stop within one day with warm clothing, food, and drink. (4) For disease on the left, prick the right; for disease on the right, prick the left. (5) The disease will stop immediately. If it does not stop, repeat the pricking with the same method.

Note:

    * Identified as Zú Qiào Yīn 足竅陰 (GB-44).

Line 18

(一) 邪客於足少陰之絡，令人嗌痛不可內食，無故善怒，氣上走賁上 。(二) 刺足下中央之脈，各三痏，凡六刺立已 。(三) 左刺右，右刺左 。(四) 嗌中腫，不能內唾，時不能出唾者，刺然骨之前出血，立已 。(五) 左刺右，右刺左 。

(1) If the evil lodges in the network vessels of the foot shàoyīn [vessel], it causes the person to suffer from pain in the throat and inability to take in food, tendency to anger without any cause, and qì ascending to above the cardia. (2) Prick the vessel in the center on the bottom of the foot,[1] three times on each side to a total of six prickings, and [the disorder] will stop immediately. (3) For disease on the left, prick the right; for disease on the right, prick the left. (4) If there is swelling inside the throat and inability to swallow down saliva and occasionally also inability to spit out saliva, prick in front of the blazing bone,[2] drawing blood, and [the disorder] will stop immediately. (5) For disease on the left, prick the right; for disease on the right, prick the left.

Notes:

    1. Identified as Yǒng Quán 湧泉 (KI-1).
    2. See the note above under line 6, same chapter on *Rán Gǔ*.

Line 19

(一) 邪客於足太陰之絡，令人腰痛引少腹控䏚眇，不可以仰息 。(二) 刺腰尻之解，兩胂之上，是腰俞 。(三) 以月死生為痏數 。發針立已 。(四) 左刺右，右刺左 。

(1) If the evil lodges in the network vessels of the foot tàiyīn [vessel], it causes the person to suffer from lumbar pain stretching to the lesser abdomen and the empty space below the rib-sides and from inability to raise the chest and breathe. (2) Prick where the lumbus and spine divide, on top of both buttocks. This is the lumbus transport point. (3) Determine the number of prickings by the waxing and waning of the

moon. As soon as you lift the needle, [the disease] will stop. (4) For disease on the left, prick the right; for disease on the right, prick the left.

Line 20

(一)邪客於足太陰之絡，令人拘攣背急，引脅而痛 。(二)刺之從項始，數脊椎俠脊，疾按之，應手如痛 。(三)刺之傍三痏，立已 。

(1) If the evil lodges in the network vessels of the foot tàiyīn [vessel], it causes the person to suffer from hypertonicity and tautness in the back, stretching into the rib-sides and causing pain. (2) Prick it starting from the nape of the neck, counting down the vertebrae on both sides of the spine, pushing down hard and responding with the hand to where [the patient] feels pain. (3) Prick next to there three times, and [the disease] will stop immediately.

Line 21

(一)邪客於足少陽之絡，令人留於樞中痛，髀不可舉 。(二)刺樞中以毫針，寒則久留針，以月死生為數，立已 。

(1) If the evil lodges in the network vessels of the foot shàoyáng [vessel], it causes the person to suffer from chronic pain in Shū Zhōng (GB-30)[1] and inability to lift the thigh. (2) Prick Shū Zhōng (GB-30) with a fine needle, in cases of cold leaving the needle in for a long time, determining the number [of prickings] by the waxing and waning of the moon, and [the disorder] will stop immediately.

Note:

* Literally meaning "center of the pivot," this is an alternate name for Huán Tiào 環跳.

Line 22

(一)治諸經，刺之 。(二)所過者不病，則繆刺之 。

(1) To treat [disease in] the various channels, prick it [directly]. (2) If the areas through which the channel passes do not show any disease,* then use the misleading pricking method to prick it.

Note:

    * I.e., the areas affected by the vessel do not show any pathologic changes, which indicates that the evil is in fact located in the network vessels instead of the main channels.

Line 23

(一)耳聾，刺手陽明 。(二)不已，刺其通脈出耳前者 。(三)齒齲，刺手陽明 。(四)不已，刺其脈入齒中者，立已 。

(1) For deafness, prick the hand yángmíng [vessel]. (2) If [the deafness] does not stop, prick the place where the vessel emerges in front of the ear.* (3) For dental cavities, prick the hand yángmíng [vessel]. (4) If [the cavities] do not stop, prick the place where the vessel enters the teeth, and it will stop immediately.

Note:

    * Identified as either Tīng Gōng 聽宮 (SI-19) or Tīng Huì 聽會 (GB-2).

Line 24

(一)邪客於五臟之間，其病也脈引而痛，時來時止 。(二)視其病，繆刺之於手足爪甲上 。(三)視其脈，出其血，間日一刺 。(四)一刺不已，五刺已 。

(1) If the evil has intruded into the space between the five viscera, such a disease also spreads along the vessels and causes pain accordingly, now coming now stopping.[1] (2) Observe the disease and prick it by the misleading pricking technique above the

finger-and toenails. (3) Observe the vessels and draw blood[2] from them, one prick-ing every other day. (4) If the disorder does not stop after one pricking, it will stop after five prickings.

Notes:

1. In this chapter and most obviously perhaps in this group of lines, it is interesting to note that *bìng* 病, which I translate literally as "disease," is seen as an actual entity that can move around in the body and spread from one channel to another, manifesting in different locations that are related to the channel it is affecting. By observing the specific symptoms, you can determine the channel that the disease is located in and then stop the disease by needling it in that channel.

2. I.e., in accordance with the findings of your visual examinations, or in other words, in relation to the state of fullness or vacuity in the vessel.

Line 25

(一)繆傳引上齒，齒唇寒痛，視其手背 。(二)脈血者去之 。(三)足陽明中指爪甲上，一痏，手大指次指爪甲上，各一痏，立已 。(四)左取右，右取左 。

(1) If [the disease] has misleadingly spread to the upper teeth,[1] manifesting in cold pain in the teeth and lips, observe the back of the hand. (2) If there is blood in the vessel [on the back of the hand], remove it.[2] (3) Prick the foot yángmíng [vessel] above the toenail of the middle toe[3] once, and above the fingernail of the thumb and index finger,[4] once each, and the disease will stop immediately. (4) For disease on the left, prick the right; for disease on the right, prick the left.

Notes:

1. Most likely meaning that the evil has moved from the hand yángmíng vessel to the foot yángmíng vessel, which exits in the upper teeth.

2. This phrase could either mean simply to remove the blood from the vessel on the back of the hand, or it could refer more generally to removing the disease, that is, the evil that has spread to the foot yángmíng vessel. In that case, the following sentence specifies the technique for doing so, thereby curing the patient.

3. Identified as Lì Duì 厲兌 (ST 45).

4. Identified as Shāng Yáng 商陽 (LI-1).

Line 26

(一)邪客於手足少陰、太陰、足陽明之絡，此五絡，皆會於耳中，上絡左額角，五絡俱竭令人身脈皆動，而形無知也。(二)其狀若尸，或曰尸厥。(三)刺足大指內側爪甲上，去端如韭葉。(四)後刺足心，後刺足中指爪甲上，各一痏，後刺少商、少衝、神門。(五)不已，以竹管吹其兩耳，剃其左角之髮方一寸燔治，飲以美酒一杯，立已。

(1) If the evil has intruded into the network vessels of the hand or foot shàoyīn, tàiyīn, or foot yángmíng [vessels], because these five [groups of] network vessels all meet inside the ear and then rise to connect to the corner of the left forehead, exhaustion in all of these five network vessels causes stirring of all the vessels in the person's body and lack of awareness of the physical body. (2) Such a patient's appearance is corpse-like, and [this disease] is sometimes referred to as corpse reversal. (3) Prick the point above the nail on the inside of the large toe, about the breadth of a leaf of Chinese chives down from the end of the nail.[1] (4) Afterwards prick the center of the foot,[2] then above the nail of the middle toe,[3] one pricking each. Then prick Shào Shāng (LU-11), Shào Chōng (HT-9), and Shén Mén (HT-7). (5) If the patient does not recover, use a bamboo tube to blow air into both ears, then shave a square *cùn* of hair from the patient's left forehead and char it. Have the patient drink it in one cup of good liquor, and immediate recovery will ensue.

Notes:

1. Identified as Yǐn Bái 隱白 (SP-1).
2. Identified as Yǒng Quán 湧泉 (KI-1).
3. Identified as Lì Duì 厲兌 (ST-45), by some commentators, even though the modern point Lì Duì is located not on the middle toe but on the second toe.

Line 27

(一)凡刺之數，先視其經脈，切而從之。(二)審其虛實而調之。(三)不調者，經刺之。(四)有痛而經不病者，繆刺之。(五)因視其皮部有血絡者，盡取之，此繆刺之數也。

(1) Whenever [you want to determine] the number of prickings, first observe the patient's vessels, palpate them and act accordingly. (2) Examine the patient's state of vacuity or repletion and regulate it. (3) If it is out of balance, use channel pricking.[1] (4) If there is pain but no signs of disease in the channels, use misleading pricking.

(5) **As you see network vessels full of blood in the layer of the skin, take these [and prick them] completely.[2] This is [how you determine] the number of misleading pricking."**

Notes:

    1. See following chapter.

    2. I.e., if you see blood stasis in any of the superficial vessels, needle them to draw out all the static blood.

針
灸
大
成
·
卷
之
一

I.17 On Channel Pricking
Jīng cì lùn
經刺論

Line 1

(一)岐伯曰：夫邪之客於形也，必先舍於皮毛 。(二)留而不去，入於孫脈，留而不去，入於絡脈，留而不去，入於經脈 。(三)內連五臟，散於腸胃，陰陽俱盛，五臟乃傷 。(四)此邪之彼皮毛而入，極於五臟之次也 。

(1) Qíbó said: "The way in which evil intrudes into the physical body is invariably by first abiding in the skin and body hair. (2) When it lodges there and is not removed, it enters the ancestral vessels. When it lodges there and is not removed, it enters the network vessels. When it lodges there and is not removed, it enters the channels. (3) Internally, it links to the five viscera and scatters in the stomach and intestines. Yīn and yáng are both exuberant and the five viscera are thereby damaged. (4) This is the order in which evil enters through the skin and body hair and ultimately ends up in the five viscera.

Line 2

(一)如此則治其經焉 。(二)凡刺之數，先視其經脈，切而從之，審其虛實而調之 。(三)不調者，經刺之 。(四)不盛不虛，以經取之 。

(1) If [a patient presents with a condition] like this, treat the patient's channels for this evil. (2) Whenever [you want to determine] the number of prickings, first observe the patient's channels, take the pulse and act accordingly, examine [the body's state of] vacuity or repletion, and regulate it. (3) If it is out of balance, [treat it by] channel pricking. (4) If it is neither exuberant nor vacuous, use the channels to take it."*

Note:

    * The meaning of this sentence is unclear, which is why I have chosen to simply translate it literally. "Take it" could be understood in the sense of "remove the evil," thereby treating the disease.

I.18 On Grand Pricking
Jù cì lùn
巨刺論

Line 1

巨刺，刺經脈；繆刺，刺絡脈。所以別也。

In [the technique of] grand pricking, prick the channels. In [the technique of] misleading pricking, prick the network vessels. This is the difference between [these two techniques].

Line 2

(一)岐伯曰：痛在於左，而右脈病者，則巨刺之。(二)邪客於經，左盛則右病，右盛則左病。(三)亦有移易者，左痛未已，而右脈先病。(四)如此者，必巨刺之，必中其經，非絡脈也。

(1) **Qíbó said:** "If the pain is on the left but the pulse on the right side reflects disease, then [treat it] with grand pricking. (2) As evil intrudes into the channels, exuberance in the left results in disease in the right, exuberance in the right results in disease in the left. (3) Moreover, there are also conditions that have a tendency to move around, where the pain on the left has not yet stopped but the pulse on the right first reflects disease. (4) If [the patient presents with a condition] like this, you must [treat the patient] with grand pricking. You must hit the channels and not the network vessels."

I.19 On the Flow of Yīn and Yáng in the Hands and Feet
Shǒu zú yīn yáng liú zhù lùn
手足陰陽流注論

Line 1

岐伯曰：凡人兩手足，各有三陰脈，三陽脈，以合為十二經也 。

Qíbó said: "All humans have two hands and two feet. In each of these, there are three yīn vessels and three yáng vessels, which combine to a total of twelve channels.

Line 2

(一)手之三陰，從胸走至手;手之三陽，從手走至頭 。(二)足之三陽，從頭下走至足;足之三陰，從足上走入腹 。(三)絡脈傳注，周流不息 。(四)故經脈者，行血氣，通陰陽，以榮於身者也 。

(1) The three yīn vessels of the hand run from the chest to the hand. The three yáng vessels of the hand run from the hand to the head. (2) The three yáng vessels of the foot run down from the head to the foot. The three yīn vessels of the foot run upwards from the foot into the abdomen. (3) The network vessels spread out and pour [their contents] everywhere without stopping. (4) Thus the channels move blood and qì and promote the flow of yīn and yáng, thereby making the body luxuriant.

Line 3

(一)其始從中焦，注手太陰 、陽明 。(二)陽明注足陽明 、太陰 。(三)太陰注手少陰 、太陽 。(四)太陽注足太陽 、少陰 。(五)少陰注手心主 、少陽 。(六)少陽注足少陽 、厥陰 。(七)厥陰復還注手太陰 。

(1) They[1] start out from the center burner and pour into the hand tàiyīn and yángmíng vessels. (2) From the [hand] yángmíng vessel, they pour into the foot yángmíng and tàiyīn vessels. (3) From the [foot] tàiyīn vessel, they pour into the hand shaoyin and tàiyáng vessels. (4) From the [hand] tàiyáng vessel, they pour into the foot tàiyáng and shàoyīn vessels. (5) From the [foot] shàoyīn vessel, they pour into

the hand heart ruler[2] and shàoyáng vessels. (6) From the shàoyáng vessel, they pour into the foot shàoyáng and juéyīn vessels. (7) From the [foot] juéyīn vessel, they return to pour back into the hand tàiyīn vessel.

Notes:

1. I.e., the content of the channels. In other texts such as *Nàn Jīng* 23, this progression refers more specifically to the flow of qì, which is naturally followed by the blood.

2. The hand heart ruler is an alternate name for the hand juéyīn [pericardium] channel. This equation is confirmed by *Líng Shū* 15, which describes the progression of circulation in the channels in almost identical words but has "hand juéyīn" here instead of "hand heart ruler."

Line 4

其氣常以平旦為紀，以漏水下百刻，晝夜流行，與天同度，終而復始也 。

The qì [in the vessels][1] invariably takes daybreak as the main thread.[2] Like water in a water clock dripping down a hundred markings, it flows day and night in measures [of time] identical to those of heaven. When finished, it begins anew.

Notes:

1. This line is a paraphrase of *Líng Shū* 76, "Movement of Defense Qì." There, the subject is defense qì.

2. I.e. organizing principle to mark its progression.

Line 5

(一)絡脈者，本經之旁支而別出，以聯絡於十二經者也 。(二)本經之脈，由絡脈而交他經，他經之交亦由是焉 。(三)傳注周流，無有停息也 。(四)夫十二經之有絡脈，猶江漢之有沱潛也 。(五)絡脈之傳注於他經，猶沱潛之旁導於他水 。

(1) The network vessels are the side branches of the root channels and emerge separately. They tie the twelve channels together into a network. (2) The vessels of the

root channels intersect with other channels by means of the network vessels, which in turn then intersect in the same way with other channels. (3) They spread out and pour [their contents] everywhere without stopping. (4) Now twelve channels having network vessels is just like the river Hàn having hidden side streams. (5) The way in which the network vessels spread out to pour into other channels resembles the way in which the hidden side streams lead to the side into other bodies of water.

Line 6

(一)是以手太陰之支者，從腕後出次指端，而交於手陽明。(二)手陽明之支者，從缺盆上俠口鼻，而交於足陽明。(三)足陽明之支者，別跗上出大指端，而交於足太陰。(四)足太陰之支者，從胃別上膈注心中，而交於手少陰。(五)手少陰則直自本經少衝穴，而交於手太陽，不假支授。蓋君者，出令者也。(六)手太陽之支者，別頰上至目內眥，而交於足太陽。(七)足太陽之支者，從膊內左右，別下合膕中，下至小指外側端，而交於足少陰；。(八)足少陰之支者，從肺出注胸中，而交於手厥陰。(九)手厥陰之支者，從掌中循小指次指出其端，而交於手少陽。(十)手少陽之支者，從耳後出至目銳眥，而交於足少陽。(十一)足少陽之支者，從跗上入大指爪甲，出三毛，而交於足厥陰。(十二)足厥陰之支者，從肝別，貫膈，上注肺，而交於手太陰也。

(1) In this way, a branch of the hand tàiyīn vessel emerges from behind the wrist by the tip of the index finger and intersects there with the hand yángmíng vessel. (2) A branch of the hand yángmíng vessel ascends from the supraclavicular fossa to "pinch"[1] the mouth and nose and intersects there with the foot yángmíng vessel. (3) A branch of the foot yángmíng vessel separates [from the main vessel] above the instep to emerge at the tip of the big toe, where it intersects with the foot tàiyīn vessel. (4) A branch of the foot tàiyīn vessel ascends from the stomach separately to the diaphragm, from where it pours into the heart and intersects with the hand shàoyīn vessel. (5) The hand shàoyīn vessel directly intersects at the Shào Chōng (HT-9) point on the root channel with the hand tàiyīn vessel, not needing to avail itself of transference by a branch. This is because it is the leader who gives orders. (6) A branch of the hand tàiyáng vessel separates [from the main channel] above the cheek to run into the inner corner of the eye, where it intersects with the foot tàiyáng vessel. (7) A branch of the foot tàiyáng vessel descends from the inside of the arm on the right and left separately to the tip of the outer edge of the little toe, where it intersects with the foot shàoyīn vessel. (8) A branch of the foot shàoyīn vessel emerges from the lung and pours into the chest, where it intersects with the hand juéyīn vessel. (9) A branch of the hand juéyīn vessel circles from the center of the palm to the little finger and the next finger at whose tip it emerges and intersects with the hand shàoyáng vessel.

(10) A branch of the hand shàoyáng vessel emerges from behind the ear and runs to the outer canthus of the eye, where it intersects with the foot shàoyáng vessel. (11) A branch of the foot shàoyáng vessel ascends from the instep, enters the nail of the big toe, and emerges at the "three hairs,"[2] where it intersects with the foot juéyīn vessel. (12) A branch of the foot juéyīn vessel separates [from the main channel] at the liver, passes through the diaphragm, and ascends to pour into the lung, where it intersects with the hand tàiyīn vessel.

Notes:

1. "Pinch" here describes the course of the network vessel, which ascends right along-side the mouth and nose.
2. *Sān máo* 三毛: Lit. "three hairs," this refers to the area where fine hair grows on top of the big toe.

Line 7

(一) 自寅時起，一晝夜，人之榮衛則以五十度周於身 。(二) 氣行一萬三千五百息，脈行八百一十丈 。(三) 運行血氣，流通陰陽，晝夜流行，與天同度，終而復始也 。

(1) Starting in the *yín* period,[1] in one day and night a person's construction and defense [qì] thus circulate through the body in 50 measures [of time each].[2] (2) [In one complete cycle], qì moves in 13,500 breaths and the vessels traverse [a distance of] 810 *zhàng*. (3) They transport blood and qì and promote the free flow of yīn and yáng. The flow continues day and night, in measures [of time] identical to those of heaven. When finished, it begins anew."

Notes:

1. *Yín shí* 寅時: the time between 3 and 5 a.m., i.e. daybreak.
2. This refers to markings of a water clock. As already mentioned above, a complete cycle of qì through the body takes exactly the same amount of time as a whole day and night, or 100 markings on the water clock.

I.20 On the Movement of Defense Qì*
Wèi qì xíng lùn
衛氣行論

Note:

    * *Líng Shū* 76, *Wèi qì xíng* 衛氣行 (The Movement of Defense Qì).

Line 1

黃帝問曰：衛氣之在於身也，上下往來不以期。候氣而刺之奈何？

The Yellow Emperor said: "As for the movement of defense qì in the body, its ascent and descent and coming and going does not occur in regular phases. How do you go about determining [the state/location of] qì before pricking?"

Line 2

(一)伯高曰：分有多少，日有長短，春秋冬夏，各有分理。(二)然後常以平旦為紀，以夜盡為始。(三)是故一日一夜，水下百刻，二十五刻者，半日之度也。常如是無已。

(1) Qíbó said: "Divisions can be many or few, days can be long or short. Spring and autumn, winter and summer, each has its principle of division. (2) This may be so, but we can invariably take daybreak as the main thread [to mark cycles of time] and the end of night as the beginning.* (3) For this reason, in one day and one night, water drips down a hundred markings [in a water clock], and 25 markings are hence the measure of half a day. This is a constant that occurs without stopping.

Note:

    * The rise of the sun signifies the beginning of the yáng aspect in nature and, in the human body, the beginning of the period when defense qì is in the yáng aspect.

Line 3

(一)日入而止，隨日之長短，各以為紀而刺之，謹候其時，病可與期。(二)失時反候者，百病不治。(三)故曰：刺實者，刺其來也。刺虛者，刺其去也。(四)此言氣存亡之時，以候虛實而刺之。

(1) Take the entering and stopping of the sun in accordance with the length of daylight* as the main thread [to mark the cycle of qì] and prick [accordingly]. If you carefully determine your timing, the disease can be [treated] in the [perfect] stage. (2) But if you lose the timing and go against [the principle of] examining [qì], you will not be able to treat any of the hundred diseases. (3) Therefore it is said: 'To prick [conditions of] repletion, prick when [qì] is arriving. To prick vacuity, prick when [qì] is leaving.' (4) This saying means that the time when qì is gathering or perishing should be used to determine [the treatment of] vacuity and repletion and you should then prick accordingly.

Note:

* In other words, calculate the progression of qì in the human body in accordance with the lengthening and shortening of daytime, which varies by the season.

Line 4

(一)是故謹候氣之所在而刺之，是謂逢時。(二)病在於三陽，必候其氣在於陽而刺之。(三)病在於三陰，必候其氣在陰分而刺之。

(1) For this reason, carefully determine where qì is at and prick only afterwards. This is what is called 'meeting the time'. (2) When the disease is in the three yáng [vessels], you must wait until the patient's qì is in yáng and only prick then. (3) When the disease is in the three yīn [vessels], you must wait until the patient's qì is in the yīn aspect and only prick afterwards.

Line 5

(一)水下一刻，人氣在太陽；水下二刻，氣在少陽；水下三刻，氣在陽明 。(二)水下四刻，氣在陰分；水下五刻，氣在太陽；水下六刻，氣在少陽；水下七刻，氣在陽明 。(三)水下八刻，氣在陰分；水下九刻，氣在太陽；水下十刻，氣在少陽；水下十一刻，氣在陽明 。(四)水下十二刻，氣在陰分；水下十三刻，氣在太陽；水下十四刻，氣在少陽；水下十五刻，氣在陽明 。(五)水下十六刻，氣在陰分；水下十七刻，氣在太陽；水下十八刻，氣在少陽；水下十九刻，氣在陽明 。(六)水下二十刻，氣在陰分；水下二十一刻，氣在太陽；水下二十二刻，氣在少陽；水下二十三刻，氣在陽明 。(七)水下二十四刻，氣在陰分；水下二十五刻，氣在太陽 。(八)此半日之度也 。

(1) As water drips down the first marking,* a person's qì is in tàiyáng. As water drips down the second marking, qì is in shàoyáng. As water drips down the third marking, qì is in yángmíng. (2) As water drips down the fourth marking, qì is in the yīn aspect. As water drips down the fifth marking, qì is in tàiyáng. As water drips down the sixth marking, qì is in shàoyáng. As water drips down the seventh marking, qì is in yángmíng. (3) As water drips down the eighth marking, qì is in the yīn aspect. As water drips down the ninth marking, qì is in tàiyáng. As water drips down the tenth marking, qì is in shàoyáng. As water drips down the eleventh marking, qì is in yángmíng. (4) As water drips down the twelfth marking, qì is in the yīn aspect. As water drips down the thirteenth marking, qì is in tàiyáng. As water drips down the fourteenth marking, qì is in shàoyáng. As water drips down the fifteenth marking, qì is in yángmíng. (5) As water drips down the sixteenth marking, qì is in the yīn aspect. As water drips down the seventeenth marking, qì is in tàiyáng. As water drips down the eighteenth marking, qì is in shàoyáng. As water drips down the nineteenth marking, qì is in yángmíng. (6) As water drips down the twentieth marking, qì is in the yīn aspect. As water drips down the twenty-first marking, qì is in tàiyáng. As water drips down the twenty-second marking, qì is in shàoyáng. As water drips down the twenty-third marking, qì is in yángmíng. (7) As water drips down the twenty-fourth marking, qì is in the yīn aspect. As water drips down the twenty-fifth marking, qì is in tàiyáng. (8) These are the measures of half a day.

Note:

   * I.e., during the time it takes water to drip down the first marking in the water clock, beginning at sunrise. During this time, the person's defense qì moves in the tàiyáng vessel.

Line 6

(一)從房至畢一十四舍，水下五十刻，日行半度，回行一舍，水下三刻與七分刻之四 。(二)大要曰：常以日之加於宿上也，人氣在太陽，是故日行一舍，人氣行三陽，行與陰分 。(三)常如是無已，天與地同紀，紛紛捲捲，終而復始 。(四)一日一夜，水下百刻而盡矣 。

(1) In the fourteen abodes from *fáng* to *bì*,* water drips down by 50 measures and the sun travels through half the sky. As it travels back one abode, water drips down three measures and 7/4th. (2) As a rule, every time the sun moves on to the next abode, a person's qì is in tàiyáng. Hence as the sun traverses a single abode, a person's qì moves through the three yáng and on into the yīn aspect. (3) This process invariably occurs like this without stopping, with heaven and earth using the same main thread [to mark their cycles], over and over in orderly cycles, beginning anew when finished. (4) In one day and one night, water drips down a hundred markings and then it is finished."

Note:

* These are names of constellations. *Shè* 舍 (abode) here refers to the 28 "mansions" (*sù* 宿) that the sun traverses in one complete cycle in traditional Chinese astronomy.

I.21 On the Essentials of Diagnosis and the Expiration of Channels[*]
Zhěn yào jīng zhōng lùn
診要經終論

Note:

[*] Excerpted from *Sù Wèn* 16, *Zhěn yào jīng zhōng lùn* 診要經終論 (On the Essentials of Diagnosis and the Expiration of Channels).

Line 1

黃帝問曰：診要何如？

The Yellow Emperor said: "What are the essentials of diagnosis?"

Line 2

(一)岐伯對曰：正月二月，天氣始方，地氣始發，人氣在肝 。(二)三月、四月，天氣正方，地氣定發，人氣在脾 。(三)五月、六月，天氣盛，地氣高，人氣在頭 。(四)七月、八月，陰氣始殺，人氣在肺 。(五)九月、十月，陰氣始冰，地氣始閉，人氣在心 。(六)十一月、十二月，冰復，地氣合，人氣在腎 。

(1) Qíbó answered: "In the first and second month, the qì of heaven is just beginning to be present and the qì of earth is beginning to rise. The person's qì is in the liver. (2) In the third and fourth month, the qì of heaven is fully there and the qì of earth is firmly risen. The person's qì is in the spleen. (3) In the fifth and sixth month, the qì of heaven is abundant and the qì of earth is high. The person's qì is in the head. (4) In the seventh and eighth month, yīn qì is beginning to kill. The person's qì is in the lung. (5) In the ninth and tenth month, yīn qì is beginning to freeze and the qì of earth is beginning to close up. The person's qì is in the heart. (6) In the eleventh and twelfth month, there is ice and concealment,[*] and the qì of earth is shut tightly. The person's qì is in the kidney.

Note:

> * While one commentary tradition of the *Sù Wèn* interprets *fù* 復 here as *fú* 伏 (latent, hidden), another interprets it as *hòu* 厚, meaning "thick, deep."

Line 3

(一)故春刺散俞，及與分理，血出而止，甚者傳氣，間者環也 。(二)夏刺絡俞，見血而止，盡氣閉環，痛病必下 。(三)秋刺皮膚，循理上下同法，神變而止 。(四)冬刺俞竅於分理，甚者直下，間者散下 。(五)春夏秋冬，各有所刺，法其所在 。

(1) For this reason, in the spring, prick the dispersed points [of the main vessels] to a depth where you reach the interstices [in the skin], drawing blood, and then stop. In severe cases, spread the qì; in light cases, [wait for] one cycle.[1] (2) In the summer, prick the points on the network vessels.[2] Stop when you see blood. Exhaust the qì and close the cycle.[3] Then the pain and disease will invariably descend. (3) In the autumn, prick the skin by following its patterns above and below in the same fashion. When you see the spirit change, stop. (4) In the winter, prick the points down to the apertures in the interstices of the seams of the flesh.[4] In severe cases, prick straight down; in light cases, go down in a scattered fashion. (5) Spring, summer, autumn, and winter, each has its own [correct way of] pricking, modeled after where qì is located.[5]

Notes:

1. According to *Sù Wèn* commentary tradition, this sentence means that, in severe cases, you should leave the needle in for a long time before removing it and, in light cases, leave the needle in until the qì has completed one revolution in the channels.
2. According to Zhāng Jièbīn, this refers to the points located on the shallow network vessels because in the summer the qì is located in the grandchild network vessels.
3. I.e., draw out all the evil qì and then close the hole by pressing down on it with your hand, so that the qì can resume its cycling. In an alternate interpretation, this last phrase could also mean to hold the hole closed for the duration of one revolution of qì in the channels.
4. Here, Zhāng Jièbīn explains that we must prick deep down in the holes between the seams of the flesh because in winter, the qì is located in the bones and marrow.

5. The information in the rest of this chapter is a summary of the *Sù Wèn* text. There, the symptoms resulting from inappropriate pricking are expanded in enough detail that commentators have been able to explain them in terms of correlative thinking and organ theory.

Line 4

(一)春刺夏分，令人不食少氣 。(二)春刺秋分，令人時驚且哭 。(三)春刺冬分，令人脹，病不愈，且欲言語 。

(1) Pricking the summer section in the spring causes the patient to suffer from lack of appetite and shortage of qì. (2) Pricking the autumn section in the spring causes the patient to suffer from intermittent fright as well as crying. (3) Pricking the winter section in the spring causes the patient to suffer from distention and, if the disease is not cured, moreover from talkativeness.

Line 5

(一)夏刺春分，令人懈惰 。(二)夏刺秋分，令人心中欲無言，惕惕如人將捕之 。(三)夏刺冬分，令人少氣，時欲怒 。

(1) Pricking the spring section in the summer causes the patient to be sluggish and lazy. (2) Pricking the autumn section in the summer causes the person to suffer in their heart from unwillingness to speak and from great fear as if there were somebody about to seize them. (3) Pricking the winter section in the summer causes the patient to suffer from shortage of qì and intermittent irascibility.

Line 6

(一)秋刺春分，令人惕然，欲有所為，起而忘之 。(二)秋刺夏分，令人嗜臥，且善夢 。(三)秋刺冬分，令人洒洒時寒 。

(1) Pricking the spring section in the autumn makes the patient fearful and wanting to do something, but only starting and then forgetting about it. (2) Pricking the summer section in the autumn causes the patient to suffer from somnolence and a tendency to dream. (3) Pricking the winter section in the autumn causes the patient

to suffer from shivering and intermittent [aversion to] cold.

Line 7

(一)冬刺春分，令人臥不能眠 。(二)冬刺夏分，令人氣上，發為諸痹 。(三)冬刺秋分，令人善渴 。

(1) Pricking the spring section in the winter causes the person to be unable to fall asleep when lying down. (2) Pricking the summer section in the winter causes the patient to suffer from qì ascent, which erupts to form the various [types] of *bì* impediment. (3) Pricking the autumn section in the winter causes the person to suffer from frequent thirst."

I.22 On Contraindications in Pricking[*]
Cì jìn lùn
刺禁論

Note:

> [*] Excerpted from *Sù Wèn* 52, *Cì jìn lùn* 刺禁論 (On Contraindications in Pricking).

Line 1

黃帝問曰：願聞禁數 。

The Yellow Emperor said: "I would like to hear about the number of contraindications. "[*]

Note:

> [*] I.e., how many locations in the body are contraindicated for being treated with acupuncture.

Line 2

岐伯曰：臟有要害，不可不察 。

Qíbó said: "Each of the viscera has places that can be injured. These must not be overlooked!

針灸大成・卷之一

Line 3

(一)肝生於左、肺藏於右、心部於表、腎治於裏、脾為之使、胃為之市。
(二)膈肓之上，中有父母；七節之旁，中有小心。

(1) The liver engenders on the left; the lung stores on the right; the heart is in charge of the exterior; the kidney governs the interior; the spleen functions as emissary; the stomach functions as the marketplace. (2) Above the diaphragm membrane, there are the father and mother[1] in the center; to the side of the seventh vertebra, there is the "small heart"[2] in the center.

Notes:

1. According to *Sù Wèn* commentaries, the "father and mother" refers to the heart and lung.
2. Different commentators interpret *xiǎo xīn* 小心 (lit. "small heart") differently. According to one school, this is a reference to the pericardium, since the "large heart" *dà xīn* 大心 refers to the heart itself. A second possible interpretation counts the seventh vertebra not from the top but in the center section of the spinal column, in which case the "small heart" is understood as referring to the kidney system, i.e. to the kidney on the left and the gate of life (*mìng mén* 命門) on the right.

Line 4

(一)從之有福，逆之有咎。(二)刺中心，一日死，其動為噫。(三)刺中肝，五日死，其動為語。(四)刺中腎，六日死，其動為嚏。(五)刺中肺，三日死，其動為欬。(六)刺中脾，十日死，其動為吞。(七)刺中膽，一日半死，其動為嘔。

(1) Observing these [contraindications] is auspicious; going against them spells disaster. (2) Hitting the heart when pricking results in death in one day. Its action will be belching.* (3) Hitting the liver when pricking results in death in five days. Its action will be speaking. (4) Hitting the kidney when pricking results in death in six days. Its action will be sneezing. (5) Hitting the lung when pricking results in death in three days. Its action will be coughing. (6) Hitting the spleen when pricking results in death in ten days. Its action will be swallowing. (7) Hitting the gallbladder when pricking results in death in one and a half days. Its action will be retching.

Note:

* I.e., The iatrogenic result of this mistake will manifest in belching.

Line 5

(一)刺足跗上中脈，血出不止，死 。(二)刺面中溜脈，不幸為盲 。(三)刺頭
中腦戶，入腦立死 。(四)刺舌下中脈太過，血出不止為瘖 。(五)刺足下布絡
中脈，血不出為腫 。(六)刺郄中大脈，令人仆脫色 。(七)刺氣街中脈，血不
出為腫鼠僕[1] 。

(1) Hitting the vessel when pricking the top of the instep results in incessant bleeding and death. (2) Hitting the vessels that flow [to the eyes] when pricking the face is inauspicious and results in blindness. (3) Hitting Nǎo Hù (GV-17)[2] when pricking the head results in immediate death if you enter the brain. (4) Hitting the vessel excessively when pricking under the tongue will cause incessant bleeding and consequently loss of voice. (5) Hitting the vessel when pricking the scattered network vessels under the foot results in swelling if there is no bleeding. (6) Hitting the large vessel when pricking Xī Zhōng causes the patient to collapse and lose all color [in the face]. (7) Hitting the vessel when pricking Qì Jiē[3] results in swelling in the groin if there is no bleeding.

Notes:

1. This is an alternate name for *shǔ xī* 鼠蹊, a technical term referring to the groin.
2. Literally, the point name translates as "window to the brain."
3. In the *Yī Zōng Jīn Jiàn* 醫宗金鑒 (Golden Mirror of Medicine) described as being located "five *cùn* below the navel and two *cùn* to both sides of the anterior median line." Also identified with Qì Chōng 氣衝 (ST-30).

Line 6

(一)刺脊間中髓為傴 。(二)刺乳上中乳房，為腫根蝕 。(三)刺缺盆中內陷，
氣泄，令人喘欬逆 。(四)刺手魚腹內陷為腫 。(五)刺陰股中大脈，血出不
止，死 。(六)刺客主人內陷中脈，為內漏，耳聾 。

(1) Hitting the marrow when pricking between the vertebrae results in bending over.[1] (2) Hitting the [inside of the breast] when pricking Rǔ Zhōng (ST-17) causes

erosion in the root of the breast. (3) Hitting and sinking in[2] when pricking Quē Pén (ST-12) causes the qì to drain and results in panting, cough, and counterflow. (4) Sinking in when pricking the fish belly of the hand[3] results in swelling. (5) Hitting the large vessel when pricking the inguinal region results in incessant bleeding and death. (6) Sinking in and hitting the vessel when pricking Kè Zhǔ Rén (GB-3) results in internal leakage[4] and deafness.

Notes:

1. I.e., a bent back.
2. I.e., inserting the needle too deeply.
3. "Fish belly of the hand" is an older name for the modern point Yú Jì 魚際 (LU-10).
4. I.e., suppuration inside the ear that subsequently leaks out.

Line 7

（一）刺膝臏，出液為跛 。（二）刺臂太陰脈，出血多，立死 。（三）刺足少陰脈，重虛出血，為舌難以言 。

(1) Pricking the knee cap so that fluid emerges will cripple the patient. (2) Pricking the hand tàiyīn vessel results in immediate death if you cause profuse bleeding. (3) Pricking the foot shàoyīn vessel, if it aggravates a [preexisting] vacuity and results in bleeding, causes the tongue to have difficulty speaking.

Line 8

（一）刺膺中陷中肺，為喘逆仰息 。（二）刺肘中內陷，氣歸之，為不屈伸 。（三）刺陰股下三寸內陷，令人遺溺 。（四）刺腋下脅間內陷，令人欬 。（五）刺少腹中膀胱，溺出，令人少腹滿 。（六）刺腨腸內陷為腫 。（七）刺眶上陷骨中脈，為漏，為盲 。（八）刺關節中液出，不得屈伸 。

(1) Sinking in and hitting the lung when pricking the center of the chest results in panting, counterflow, and bending backwards during breathing. (2) Sinking in when pricking the middle of the elbow causes the qì to return there[1] and results in inability to bend and stretch. (3) Sinking in when pricking three *cùn* below the groin causes enuresis in the patient. (4) Sinking in when pricking between the area below the

armpit and the rib-side causes coughing in the patient. (5) Hitting the bladder when pricking the lesser abdomen causes urine to leak out and results in lesser abdominal fullness in the patient. (6) Sinking in when pricking Chuǎi Cháng (BL-56)[2] results in swelling. (7) Sinking into the bone and hitting the vessel when pricking above the eye socket results in tearing and blindness. (8) Discharge of fluid when pricking the joints will result in inability to bend and stretch.

Notes:

1. In other words, wrong pricking in this area causes the qì to gather there instead of dispersing and flowing freely.
2. An alternate name for Chéng Jīn 承筋 (BL-56).

Line 9

（一）無刺大醉，令人氣亂 。（二）無刺大怒，令人氣逆 。（三）無刺大勞人，無刺新飽人，無刺大饑人，無刺大渴人，無刺大驚人 。（四）新內無刺；已刺勿內 。（五）已醉勿刺；已刺勿醉 。（六）新怒勿刺；已刺勿怒 。（七）新勞勿刺；已刺勿勞 。（八）已飽勿刺；已刺勿飽 。（九）已饑勿刺，已刺勿饑 。（十）已渴勿刺，已刺勿渴 。

(1) Do not prick a greatly intoxicated [patient]. It will cause chaotic qì in the person. (2) Do not prick a greatly angered [patient]. It will cause qì counterflow in the person. (3) Do not prick a greatly overworked person, do not prick a recently satiated person,[1] do not prick a severely starved person, do not prick a severely thirsty person, do not prick a greatly frightened person. (4) Do not prick [a patient] who has just had sexual intercourse; after pricking,[2] do not [allow the patient to] have sexual intercourse.[3] (5) Do not prick [a patient] who is already intoxicated; after pricking, do not [allow the patient to] become intoxicated. (6) Do not prick [a patient] who has just been angered. After pricking, do not [allow the patient to] become angered. (7) Do not prick [a patient] who has just been overworked; after pricking, do not [allow the patient to] become overworked. (8) Do not prick [a patient] after they have eaten to satiety; after pricking, do not [allow the patient to] eat to satiety. (9) Do not prick [a patient] who is starving; after pricking, do not [allow the patient to] starve. (10) Do not prick [a patient] who is thirsty; after pricking, do not [allow the patient to be] thirsty.

針灸大成 • 卷之一

Notes:

1. I.e., a person who has recently eaten a large meal.
2. I.e., after receiving acupuncture.
3. This and the following lines are no longer part of the *Sù Wèn* source text. The Chinese text literally says "After recent intercourse, do not prick; after pricking, do not have sexual intercourse," leaving it open whether the subject of this sentence is the acupuncturist or the patient. Nevertheless, given the previous phrase, it seems more likely that this prohibition refers to the person receiving the acupuncture, not the person administering the treatment.

Line 10

(一)乘車來者，臥而休之，如食頃乃刺 。(二)出行來者，坐而休之，如行十里乃刺之 。(三)大驚大恐，必定其氣乃刺之 。

(1) If [a patient] has arrived riding in a carriage, make them lie down and rest. Only prick them after the amount of time it takes to eat a meal. (2) If [a patient] has arrived on foot, make them sit down and rest. Only prick them after the amount of time it takes to walk ten *lǐ*. (3) If [a patient] is greatly frightened or fearful, you must stabilize the qì before pricking them."

I.23 In [Patients Suffering from] the Five Despoliations, Do not Drain[1,2]
Wǔ duó bù kě xiè
五奪不可瀉

Notes:

1. Wiseman and Feng translate *duó* 奪 (lit. "to snatch or rest") as a technical term in the medical context as "despoliate" and paraphrase this as "(of blood, fluid, or essence) to be suddenly and severely depleted" (*A Practical Dictionary of Chinese Medicine*, p. 124).
2. Excerpted from *Líng Shū* 61, *Wǔ jìn* 五禁 (The Five Contraindications).

(一)岐伯曰：形容已脫，是一奪也 。(二)夫脫血之後，是二奪也 。(三)大汗之後，是三奪也 。(四)大泄之後，是四奪也 。(五)新產大血之後，是五奪也 。(六)此皆不可瀉 。

(1) Qíbó said: "If the physical body is severely emaciated,[1] this is the first despoliation. (2) After shedding blood, this is the second despoliation. (3) After great sweating, this is the third despoliation. (4) After great diarrhea, this is the fourth despoliation. (5) After great bleeding soon after childbirth, this is the fifth despoliation. (6) In all of these [situations], you must not drain."[2]

Notes:

1. The reason for my choice of translation here is based on the slightly different source text, *Líng Shū* 61, where the line reads as follows: 形肉已奪是一奪也 。
2. Given the context here both in the present text and in *Líng Shū* 61, it is obvious that "drain" here refers to the application of acupuncture in such a way that it drains qì because the body's right qì is already weakened and depleted to such an extent that it must first be supported by supplementation. Some commentators interpret this warning as meaning that such cases should not be treated with acupuncture at all, but only with medicinal therapy. This notion is, however, not supported by the text, which merely warns against "draining."

I.24 In the Four Seasons, Do not Prick
Sì jì bù kě cì
四季不可刺

（一）岐伯曰：正月、二月、三月，人氣在左。（二）無刺左足之陽。（三）四月、五月、六月，人氣在右。（四）無刺右足之陽。（五）七月、八月、九月，人氣在右。（六）無刺右足之陰。（七）十月、十一月、十二月，人氣在左。（八）無刺左足之陰。

(1) Qíbó said: "In the first, second, and third months,* a person's qì is in the left [side of the body]. (2) Do not prick the yáng [points] of the left foot. (3) In the fourth, fifth, and sixth months, a person's qì is in the right [side of the body]. (4) Do not prick the yáng [points] of the right foot. (5) In the seventh, eighth, and ninth months, a person's qì is in the right [side of the body]. (6) Do not prick the yīn [points] of the right foot. (7) In the tenth, eleventh, and twelfth months, a person's qì is in the left [side of the body]. (8) Do not prick the yīn [points] of the left foot."

Note:

* Note that the months of the traditional Chinese calendar do not coincide with our modern months of January, February, etc., but are based on the lunar calendar. Please see volume five, Appendix B of the *Great Compendium of Acupuncture and Moxibustion*, translated by Lorraine Wilcox.

I.25 At the Time of Death, Do not Prick[*]
Sǐ qī bù kě cì
死期不可刺

Note:

[*] Excerpted from *Sù Wèn* 65, *Biāo běn bìng chuán lùn* 標本病傳論 (On the Tip and Root and on Disease Transmission).

Line 1

(一)岐伯曰：病先發於心，心主痛。(二)一日而之肺，加欬。(三)三日而之肝，加脅支痛。(四)五日而之脾，加閉塞不通，身痛體重。(五)三日不已，死。(六)冬夜半，夏日中。

(1) Qíbó said: "If disease arises first in the heart, the main symptom will be heart pain. (2) If, after one day, [the disease] passes into the lung, [the condition] will be aggravated by cough. (3) If, after three [more] days, it passes into the liver, it will be aggravated by propping pain in the rib-sides. (4) If, after five [more] days, it passes into the spleen, it will be aggravated by blockage and stoppage, and by generalized pain and heaviness. (5) If there is no recovery within three [more] days, death will ensue. (6) In the winter, [death will occur] at midnight; in the summer, at midday.

Line 2

(一)病先發於肺，喘欬。(二)三日而之肝，脅支滿痛。(三)一日而之脾，身重體痛。(四)五日而之胃，脹。(五)十日不已，死。(六)冬日入，夏日出。

(1) If disease arises first in the lung, [it will manifest in] panting and cough. (2) If, after three days, [the disease] passes into the liver, there will be propping fullness and pain in the rib-sides. (3) If, after one [more] day, it passes into the spleen, there will be generalized heaviness and pain. (4) If, after five [more] days, it passes into the stomach, there will be distention. (5) If there is no recovery within ten [more] days, death will ensue. (6) In the winter, [death will occur] at sunset; in the summer, at sunrise.

Line 3

(一)病先發於肝，頭目眩，脅支滿 。(二)三日而之脾，體重身痛 。(三)五日而之胃，脹 。(四)三日而之腎，腰脊少腹痛，脛痠 。(五)三日不已，死 。(六)冬日入，夏早食 。

(1) If disease arises first in the liver, [it will manifest in] dizziness in the head and eyes and in propping fullness in the rib-sides. (2) If, after three days, [the disease] passes into the spleen, there will be generalized heaviness and pain. (3) If, after five [more] days, it passes into the stomach, there will be distention. (4) If, after three [more] days, it passes into the kidney, there will be pain in the lumbar spine and lesser abdomen and aching lower legs. (5) If there is no recovery within three [more] days, death will ensue. (6) In the winter, [death will occur] at sunset; in the summer, at breakfast time.*

Note:

* I.e., 7-9 am.

Line 4

(一)病先發於脾，身痛體重 。(二)一日而之胃，脹 。(三)二日而之腎，少腹腰脊痛，脛痠 。(四)三日而之膀胱，背膂筋痛，小便閉 。(五)十日不已，死 。(六)冬人定，夏晏食 。

(1) If disease arises first in the spleen, [it will manifest in] generalized pain and heaviness. (2) If, after one day, it passes into the stomach, there will be distention. (3) If, after two [more] days, it passes into the kidney, there will be pain in the lesser abdomen and lumbar spine, and aching lower legs. (4) If, after three [more] days it passes into the bladder, there will be pain in the back and paravertebral sinews, and urinary block. (5) If there is no recovery within ten [more] days, death will ensue. (6) In the winter, [death will occur] between 9 and 11 pm; in the summer, during [the early] meal time.*

Note:

    * In a commentary on the *Sù Wèn*, Wáng Bīng explains these two time measurements as 25 *kè* 刻 (quarter hours) after the time of *shēn* 申 (3-5pm) and after the time of *yín* 寅 (3-5am) respectively. "[Early] meal time" is an alternative term for *zǎo shí* 早食 ("breakfast") and refers to the time from 7-9 am. The term *rén dìng* 人定 can literally be explained as the time when "human affairs are settled," in the sense that it is so late at night that people have gone to sleep.

Line 5

（一）病先發於腎，少腹腰脊痛，胻痠 。（二）三日而之膀胱，背膂筋痛，小便閉 。（三）三日而上之心，心脹 。（四）三日而之小腸，兩脅支痛 。（五）三日不已，死 。（六）冬大晨，夏晏晡 。

(1) If disease arises first in the kidney, [it will manifest in] pain in the lesser abdomen and lumbar spine, and in aching in the calves. **(2)** If, after three days, it passes into the bladder, there will be pain in the back and paravertebral sinews, as well as urinary block. **(3)** If, after three [more] days, it rises and passes into the heart, there will be distention in the heart. **(4)** If, after three [more] days, it passes into the small intestine, there will be propping pain in both rib-sides. **(5)** If there is no recovery within three [more] days, death will ensue. **(6)** In the winter, [death will occur] at dawn; in the summer, at dusk.*

Note:

    * These time markers are alternate terms for the more common names *píng dàn* 平旦 and *huáng hūn* 黃昏, which refer to 3-5 am and 7-9 pm respectively.

Line 6

（一）病先發於胃，脹滿 。（二）五日而之腎，少腹腰脊痛，胻痠 。（三）三日而之膀胱，背膂筋痛，小便閉 。（四）五日而之脾，身體重 。（五）六日不已，死 。（六）冬夜半，夏日晡 。

(1) If disease arises first in the stomach, [it will manifest in] distention and fullness. **(2)** If, after five days, it passes into the kidney, there will be pain in the lesser abdomen and lumbar spine, and soreness in the calves. **(3)** If, after three [more] days, it passes into the bladder, there will be pain in the back and paravertebral sinews, as well as urinary block. (4) If, after five [more] days, it passes into the spleen, there will be generalized heaviness. (5) If there is no recovery within six [more] days, death will ensue. (6) In the winter, [death will occur] at midnight; in the summer, in the late afternoon.*

Note:

    * I.e., 3-5 pm.

Line 7

(一)病先發於膀胱，小便閉 。(二)五日而之腎，少腹脹，腰脊痛，胻痠 。(三)一日而之小腸，肚脹 。(四)一日而之脾，身體重 。(五)二日不已，死 。(六)冬雞鳴，夏下晡 。

(1) If disease arises first in the bladder, [it will manifest in] urinary block. (2) If, after five days, it passes into the kidney, there will be lesser abdominal distention, pain in the lumbar spine, and aching in the calves. (3) If, after one [more] day, it passes into the small intestine, there will be distention in the belly. (4) If, after one [more] day, it passes into the spleen, there will be generalized heaviness. (5) If there is no recovery within two [more] days, death will ensue. (6) In the winter, [death will occur] at the time of cockcrow*; in the summer, in the late afternoon.

Note:

    * I.e., 1-3 am

Line 8

(一)諸病以次相傳 。(二)如是者，皆有死期，不可刺也 。(三)間有一臟及二三臟者，乃可刺也 。

(1) All disease is transmitted [between the viscera] according to a specific order. (2) If the order is like this,* each has a time for death, when you cannot [save the patient] by pricking. (3) If there are one or two or three viscera in between, then you can [save the patient] by pricking.

Note:

* I.e., as outlined in the preceding lines.

I.26 On Pricking Methods*
Cì fǎ lùn
刺法論

Note:

* Excerpted from *Sù Wèn* 72, *Cì fǎ lùn* 刺法論 (On Pricking Methods). This chapter is an apocryphal chapter of the *Sù Wèn* that is recorded as lost in many editions, and in others credited to Wáng Bīng as an eighth-century addition. It is part of the section in the *Sù Wèn* that discusses the doctrine of the "five movements and six qì" (*wǔ yùn liù qì* 五運六氣). The text here is loosely based on the *Sù Wèn* chapter, but contains much additional information, most notably the invocations and similar ritual actions. See also *Lèi Jīng* 類經 (Classified Classic) 44.

Line 1

(一)黃帝問曰：人虛即神遊失守位，使鬼神外干，是致夭亡。(二)何以全真？願聞刺法。

The Yellow Emperor asked: "When a person is vacuous, the spirit wanders astray and loses its guard and place, which permits demons and spirits to harass it from the outside. This then results in premature death. (2) How can you conserve the true [qì] in its completeness? I would like to hear the method of pricking [for this purpose]."

Line 2

(一)岐伯曰：神移失守，雖在其體，然不致死，或有邪干，故令夭壽。(二)只如厥陰失守，天已虛，人氣肝虛，感天重虛，即魂遊於上。(三)邪干厥陰，大氣身溫，猶可刺之。(四)刺足少陽之所過。(五)咒曰：太上元君，鬱鬱青龍，常居其左，制之三魂。誦三遍。(六)次呼三魂名：爽靈，胎光，幽精，誦三遍。(七)次想青龍於穴下。刺之。可徐徐出針，親令人按氣於

144

口中 。(八)腹中鳴者可活 。(九)次刺肝之俞 。(十)咒曰: 太微帝君，元英制魂，貞元及本，令入青雲 。(十一)又呼三魂名如前，三遍 。

(1) Qíbó said: "In cases where the spirit shifts and has lost its guard, if it is still in the person's body, it will not result in death. Alternatively, if there is [external] evil harassing it, this causes [the person's] life to be cut short. (2) For example, at a time when the juéyīn [aspect in the cosmos] has lost its guard and heaven then becomes vacuous, if the person's qì becomes vacuous in the liver aspect, it is affected by heaven and the vacuity is doubled. Then the ethereal soul wanders astray upward.[1] (3) If [external] evil harasses juéyīn, if the great qì in the body is still warm, you can still [rescue the patient] by pricking.[2] (4) Prick where the foot shàoyáng [vessel] passes over.[3] (5) Invocation: 'Great Supreme Lord, Luxuriant Green Dragon who constantly sits to his left! Control the three ethereal souls!' Recite this three times! (6) Next, call out the names of the three ethereal souls: 'Shuǎnglíng, Tāiguāng, Yōujīng!' Recite three times! (7) Next, visualize the Green Dragon below the [acupuncture] point. Prick it. You can very slowly remove the needle and have another person close-by press qì into the [patient's]mouth. (8) If there are sounds in the center of the abdomen, [the patient] can survive. (9) Next, prick the liver transport points.[4] (10) Invocation: 'Lord Emperor of Great Tenuity, Primordial Hero who controls the ethereal souls, origin of rectitude who reaches the root, allow to enter the green-blue clouds.'[5] (11) Again call out the names of the three ethereal souls as before, three times![6]

Notes:

1. The commentary here adds: "If vacuity in the liver and vacuity in heaven are further complicated by sweating, this is called 'triple vacuity.' The spirit wanders astray to the top, where there is no great lord on the left and the spirit light fails to gather. The ghost White Corpse (bái shī 白尸) arrives and causes the person to die all of a sudden."
2. The commentary here adds an explanation to describe the signs when the condition is still treatable: "The eyes have spirit, the heart and abdomen are still warm, there is no saliva in the mouth, and the tongue and testicles are not contracted." The Sù Wèn passage is here slightly different: 邪干厥大氣身溫... "If [external] evil harasses, reversal of great qì will result. If the body is still warm...
3. The meaning of guò 過 is unclear here, but commentary traditions of both the Sù Wèn text and the present text paraphrase this as an instruction to prick Qiū Xū 邱墟 (GB-40).
4. The commentary here explains that these points are located below the ninth vertebra on both sides of the body.

5. As is the case in much ritual language, it is very difficult (and often futile) to try to reconstruct the meaning of old curses and invocations, since their efficacy is derived not only from the meaning but also from the precise sound of the invocation.

6. The commentary here adds the following instruction: "Prick [down] three *fēn*, leave [the needle] in for three invocations, then advance it one [additional] *fēn*, leave it in for three [additional] invocations, then reverse and pull [the needle] back two *fēn*, leave it in for one invocation, and gently remove the needle. The qì will then return [and the patient] will live."

Line 3

(一)人病心虛，又遇君相二火司天失守，感而三虛。遇火不及，黑尸鬼犯之，令人暴亡。(二)可刺手少陽之所過。(三)咒曰：太乙帝君，泥丸總神，丹無黑氣，來復其真。誦三遍。(四)想赤鳳於穴下，復刺心俞。(五)咒曰：丹房守靈，五帝上清，陽和布體，來復黃庭。誦三遍。

(1) If a person suffers from vacuity in the heart and moreover encounters [a time when] the sovereign fire or the ministerial fire controlling heaven has lost its guard, and then contracts [external evil], it is a triple vacuity.[1] [If the patient then] encounters [a year when the movement of] fire is inadequate, the Black Corpse demon will invade the person and cause him or her to perish all of a sudden.[2] (2) You can prick the place where the hand shàoyáng [vessel] passes over.[3] (3) Invocation: 'Lord Emperor of Primordial Unity, assemble the spirits in *Ní wán*.[4] In cinnabar, there is no black qì. Come and return to your true [place]!' Recite this three times! (4) Visualize the red phoenix below the point, then prick the heart transport points.[5] (5) Invocation: 'In the cinnabar house, guard the spirits and the five emperors in upper clarity. May yáng warmth spread through the body. Come and return to the yellow court!' Recite this three times!

Notes:

1. The commentary to *Sù Wèn* 72 here explains "triple vacuity" as being caused by "vacuity of the person's qì, combined with vacuity of heaven's qì, and then compounded by encountering fright, which despoliates the essence, causing sweating in the heart."

2. Because of the complexities of the doctrine of "five movements and six qì" and the apocryphal nature of this chapter already in the *Sù Wèn*, the meaning of this line is unclear and the translation here is questionable, based on the commentary to *Sù Wèn* 72, as well as on more complete similar versions in the following lines. The color of the invading demon, black, is associated with water, which in the order of conquest in the

five phases, conquers fire.

3. Again, the meaning of "passes over" is unclear, but the commentary tradition to *Sù Wèn* 72 associates this description with Yáng Chí 陽池 (TB-4) and adds that the patient is treatable if "the tongue and testicles are not contracted and the spirit in the eyes has not changed."

4. A Daoist term, referring to the most central among the nine palaces of the brain, the place where the original spirit is stored.

5. Here the commentary adds: "Prick down three *fēn*, leave [the needle] in for one breath, then again advance it one [more] *fēn*, leave it in for three [more] breaths, then pull it back, leave it in for one breath, and gently take it out. Stroke the point and this will immediately cause [the patient] to return to life." It moreover identifies the "heart transport points" as "to both sides of the fifth vertebra."

Line 4

(一)人脾病又遇太陰司天失守，感而三虛。又遇土不及，青尸鬼犯之，令人暴亡。(二)可刺足陽明之所過。(三)咒曰：常在魂庭，始清太寧，元和布氣，六甲及真。誦三遍。(四)先想黃庭於穴下，復刺脾俞。(五)咒曰：大始乾位，總統坤元，黃庭真氣，來復遊全。誦三遍。

(1) If a person suffers from spleen disease and moreover encounters a time when tàiyīn controlling heaven has lost its guard, and then contracts [external evil], it is a triple vacuity. [If the patient then] encounters [a year when the movement of] earth is inadequate, the Green-Blue Corpse demon will invade the person and cause him or her to perish all of a sudden. (2) You can prick the place where the foot yángmíng [vessel] passes over.[1] (3) Invocation: 'Always in the court of the ethereal soul, initial purity and great tranquility, original warmth, spread the qì, in the six *jiǎ* times[2] reach perfection.' Recite this three times! (4) First visualize the yellow court below the point, then prick the spleen transport points.[3] (5) Invocation: 'Great beginning in the position of *qián*, total control in the origin of *kūn*,[4] true qì of the yellow court, come and return to complete your wandering.' Recite this three times![5]

Notes:

1. In the commentary identified as Chōng Yáng 衝陽 (ST-42).

2. A reference to the stems and branches system of counting time in traditional Chinese culture.

3. The commentary here instructs before pricking the spleen transport points to "insert the needle three [*fēn*], leave it in for three [breaths], then advance it another two [*fēn*], leave it in for one breath, very gently remove it, and stroke [the point] with the hand." It also describes the spleen transport points as being located "below the eleventh vertebra, on both sides."

4. *Qián* and *kūn* are two of the eight trigrams from the *Book of Changes*.
5. The commentary here adds: "Prick three [*fēn*] down, leave [the needle] in for two [breaths], advance [another] five [*fēn*]. When the stirring qì arrives, gently remove the needle."

Line 5

(一)人肺病，遇陽明同天失守，感而三虛，又遇金不及，有赤尸鬼干人，令人暴亡。(二)可刺手陽明之所過。(三)咒曰：青氣真全，帝符日元，七魂歸右，今復本田。誦三遍。(四)想白虎於穴下，復刺肺俞。(五)咒曰：左元真人，六合氣賓，天符帝力，來入其門。誦三遍。

(1) If a person suffers from lung disease and moreover encounters a time when yáng-míng controlling heaven has lost its guard, and then contracts [external evil], it is a triple vacuity. [If the patient then] encounters [a year when the movement of] metal is inadequate, the Red Corpse demon will invade the person and cause him or her to perish all of a sudden. (2) You can prick the place where the hand yángmíng [vessel] passes over.[1] (3) Invocation: 'Green-blue qì of true completeness, imperial talisman for the origin of the sun, may the seven ethereal souls return to the right, now return to your original field.' Recite this three times! (4) Visualize the white tiger below the point, and then prick the transport points of the lung.[2] (5) Invocation: 'Perfected person in the left origin, I pay respect to the qì of the six directions, heavenly talisman with imperial strength. Come and enter its gate!' Recite three times.[3]

Notes:

1. In the commentary identified with Hé Gǔ 合谷 (LI-4).
2. The commentary here instructs the reader, before pricking the lung transport points, to "insert the needle three [*fēn* down], leave it in for three [breaths], then advance it two [more *fēn*], leave it in for three [breaths], then pull it back, leave it in for one [more breath], gently remove it, and stroke [the point]." It furthermore describes the lung transport points as being located "below the third vertebra on both sides."
3. The commentary here adds: "Insert the needle one and a half [*fēn*], leave it in for three breaths, then advance it another two [*fēn*], leave it in for one more breath, then gently remove it and stroke [the point] with the hand."

Line 6

（一）人腎病，又遇太陽司天失守，感而三虛，又遇水運不及之年，有黃尸鬼干人正氣，吸人神魂，致暴亡。（二）可刺足太陽之所過。（三）咒曰：元陽盲嬰，五老及真，泥丸玄華，補精長存。（四）想黑氣於穴下，復刺腎俞。（五）咒曰：天玄日晶，太和昆靈，貞元內守，待入始清。誦三遍。

(1) If a person suffers from kidney disease and moreover encounters a time when tàiyáng controlling heaven has lost its guard, and then contracts [external evil], this is a triple vacuity. [If the patient then] encounters a year when the movement of water is inadequate, the Yellow Corpse demon will invade the person's right qì and suck in the person's spirit and ethereal souls, causing him or her to perish all of a sudden. (2) You can prick the place where the foot tàiyáng [vessel] passes over.[1] (3) Invocation: "Blind infant of original yáng, five elders reaching perfection, profound florescence of *Ní wán*, supplement the essence and give long life!" (4) Visualize black qì below the point, and then prick the kidney transport points.[2] (5) Invocation: "Heaven's profundity and sun's brilliance, grand harmony for the spirits of posterity, origin of rectitude, guard on the inside, wait and enter beginning purity!" Recite this three times!"[3]

Notes:

1. In the commentary identified as Jīng Gǔ 京骨 (BL-64).
2. The commentary here instructs before pricking the kidney transport points to "insert the needle one and a half [*fēn*], leave it in for three breaths, advance it three [*fēn*], leave it in for one breath, gently remove the needle, and stroke the point." It further describes the kidney transport points as being located "below the fourteenth vertebra, on both sides."
3. The commentary adds: "Insert the needle three *fēn*, leave in for three breaths, advance three *fēn*, leave in for three breaths, then remove the needle very gently and stroke the point."

I.27 On the Correspondence of the Five Pricking Methods to the Five Viscera*
Wǔ cì yīng wǔ zàng lùn
五刺應五臟論

Note:

* Excerpted from *Líng Shū* 7, *Guān zhēn* 官針 (Using Needles).

Line 1

岐伯曰：凡刺有五，以應五臟 。

Qíbó said: "There are five [methods of] pricking, corresponding to the five viscera.

Line 2

(一) 一曰半刺者：淺內而疾發，無針肉，如拔毛狀，以取皮氣，以應肺
也 。(二) 二曰豹文刺者：左右前後針之，中脈，以取經絡之血，以應心
也 。(三) 三曰關刺者：直刺左右盡筋上，以取筋痹，慎無出血，以應肝
也 。(四) 四曰合谷刺者：左右雞足，針於分肉之間，以取肌痹，以應脾
也 。(五) 五曰輸刺者：直入直出，深內至骨，以取骨痹，以應腎也 。

(1) The first method is called 'half pricking.' [In this method,] insert the needle shallowly and remove it quickly. Do not needle the flesh. [Needle] as if you were pulling out a hair. Use [this method] to remove qì from the skin. It corresponds to the lung. (2) The second method is called 'leopard pattern pricking.' [In this method, insert] the needle [to the right and left and front and back, in the middle of the vessels. Use [this method] to remove blood from the channels and network vessels. It corresponds to the heart. (3) The third method is called 'joint pricking.' [In this method,] prick straight down to the right and left [of the joints], on top of the ends of the sinews. Use [this method] to remove impediment from the sinews. Be careful not to draw blood. It corresponds to the liver. (4) The fourth method is called 'valley-closing pricking.'[1] [In this method, insert the needle] to the left and right [in a pattern

150

that resembles] chicken feet.[2] Needle in the space of the seams of the flesh. Use [this method] to remove impediment from the flesh. It corresponds to the spleen. (5) The fifth method is called 'transport pricking.' [In this method,] enter and exit straight, [prick] deeply down to the inside until you reach the bones. Use [this method] to remove impediment from the bones. It corresponds to the kidney."

Notes:

1. Note that in this case, *hé gǔ* 合谷 does not refer to the point Hé Gǔ 合谷 (LI-4) on the Large Intestine Channel, but is a technical term to describe this needling method.
2. I.e., in a pattern that looks like a "Y," by inserting the needle obliquely from the center to the right and left sides.

I.28 On the Correspondence of the Nine Pricking Methods to the Nine Transformations[*]
Jiǔ cì yīng jiǔ biàn lùn
九刺應九變論

Note:

[*] Excerpted from *Líng Shū* 7, *Guān zhēn* 官針 (Using Needles).

Line 1

岐伯曰：凡刺有九，以應九變 。

Qíbó said: "There are nine methods of pricking, corresponding to the nine transformations."

Line 2

（一）一曰輸刺者：諸經滎輸臟俞也 。（二）二曰遠道刺者：病在上，取之下，刺腑俞也 。（三）三曰經刺者：刺大經之結絡經分也 。（四）四曰絡刺者：刺者，刺小絡，血脈也 。（五）五曰分刺者：刺分肉間也 。（六）六曰大瀉刺者：刺大膿也 。（七）七曰毛刺者：刺浮皮毛也 。（八）八曰巨刺者：左取右，右取左也 。（九）九曰焠刺者：燔針，以取痺也 。

(1) The first one is called 'transport pricking'. [In this method,] prick the various channels at the brook points and the transport points of the viscera. (2) The second one is called 'distant-path pricking'. [In this method,] the disease is on top but you remove it by [pricking] below. Prick the bowel points. (3) The third one is called 'channel pricking'. [In this method,] prick the seams between the channels and network vessels where the major channels are tied together. (4) The fourth one is called 'network vessel pricking'. [In this method,] prick the minor network vessels, which are the [shallow] blood vessels. (5) The fifth one is called 'seams pricking'. [In this method,] prick in the seams between the flesh. (6) The sixth one is called 'great draining pricking'. [Use this method to] prick major [accumulations of] pus. (7) The

seventh one is called 'hair pricking'. [In this method,] prick superficially in the [area of the] skin and body hair. (8) The eighth one is called 'grand pricking'. For [disease] on the left, take [points] on the right; for [disease] on the right, take [points] on the left. (9) The ninth one is called 'red-hot pricking'. Heat the needle until it is glowing red. Use [this method] to remove impediment."

I.29 On the Correspondence of the Twelve Pricking Methods to the Twelve Channels*
Shí èr cì yīng shí èr jīng lùn
十二刺應十二經論

Note:

* Excerpted from *Líng Shū* 7, *Guān zhēn* 官針 (Using Needles).

Line 1

岐伯曰：凡刺有十二，以應十二經。

Qíbó said: "There are twelve methods of pricking, corresponding to the twelve channels.

Line 2

(一)一曰偶刺者：以手直心若背，直痛所，一刺前，一刺後，以治心痹。
(二)二曰報刺者：刺痛無常處，上下行者。直內無拔針，以手隨病所按
之，乃出針復刺也。(三)三曰恢刺者：直刺傍，舉之前後，恢筋急，以治筋
痹。(四)四曰齊刺者：直入一，旁入二，以寒氣少深者。(五)五曰揚刺者
：正內一，旁內四，而浮之，以治寒氣博大者。(六)六曰直針刺者：引皮
以刺之，以治寒氣之淺者。(七)七曰輸刺者：直入直出，稀發針而深之，
以治氣盛而熱者。(八)八曰短刺者：刺骨痹，稍遙而深之，置針骨所，以
上下摩骨也。(九)九曰浮刺者：旁入而浮之，以治肌急而寒者。(十)十曰
陰刺者：左右率刺之，以治寒厥。中寒厥，足踝後少陰也。(十一)十一曰
傍針刺者：宜傍刺各一，以治留痹久居者。(十二)十二曰贊刺者：直入直
出，數發針而淺之，出血，是謂治癰腫也。

(1) The first one is called 'paired pricking'. [In this method,] place your hand directly on the heart and on the back. [Prick] straight down where the pain is located, one prick in the front and one in the back. Use [this method] to treat heart impediment.
(2) The second one is called 'reciprocal pricking'. [With this method,] prick pain

154

that does not have a constant location but moves up and down. Prick straight to the inside [of the place where the pain is presently located] and do not pull the needle out. With your [other] hand, follow the disease [to the new location of pain] and press down there. Now remove the needle [from the old location] and then prick [the new location of pain]. (3) The third one is called 'waggling pricking'. [In this method,] prick straight down the side [of the sinew where the pain is located], lift [the sinew] in the front and in the back, and waggle the sinew [to relieve] tension. Use [this method] to treat impediment in the sinews. (4) The fourth one is called 'one-on-either-side pricking'. [In this method,] insert one needle straight down and insert two [more needles] on the side. Use [this method] to treat cold qì that is rather reduced but deep.[1] (5) The fifth one is called 'raising needling'. [In this method,] insert one needle right in the center and four [more needles] on the four sides. Prick superficially. Use [this method] to treat cold qì that is rather extensive and large.[2] (6) The sixth one is called 'straight-needle pricking'. [In this method,] pull the skin and then prick.[3] Use [this method] to treat cold qì that is shallow. (7) The seventh one is called 'point pricking'. Prick straight in and and straight back out, apply the needle only a few times but deeply.[4] Use [this method] to treat qì exuberance and heat. (8) The eighth one is called 'short pricking'. [Use this method] to prick bone impediment. Slightly shake [the needle after inserting it] and then insert it more deeply, [until] you have placed the needle where the bone is. Move it up and down to rub against the bone. (9) The ninth one is called 'shallow pricking'. Prick by entering from the side and insert it shallowly. Use [this method] to treat tension in the flesh with [aversion to] cold. (10) The tenth one is called 'yīn pricking'. [In this method,] prick both the right and left sides [simultaneously]. Use [this method] to treat cold reversal. When [a patient] is struck by cold reversal, [prick] behind the ankle on the shàoyīn [vessel].[5] (11) The eleventh one is called 'side-needle pricking'. [In this method,] it is suitable to prick once [in the center] and once its side.[6] Use [this method] to treat abiding impediment that is chronic. (12) The twelfth one is called 'assistance pricking'. Prick straight in and straight back out. Apply the needle numerous times and prick shallowly, drawing blood. This method is so-called because it treats welling-abscesses."

Notes:

1. The commentators to this line in the *Líng Shū* explain this as a type of condition where the cold is concentrated in only a small area but is deep below the surface. The *Líng Shū* also calls this method "triple needling" because you insert a total of three needles.

2. I.e., treat cold conditions that are wide-spread in their distribution throughout the body.

3. I.e., lift the skin up and insert the needle shallowly only into the skin fold, without entering the muscle.

4. According to the modern commentary to *Líng Shū* 7, this means that you only selected a limited number of major points.

5. As the commentary to *Líng Shū* 7 explains, you insert two needles at exactly the same time to the same depth, one with the right hand and one with the left hand, at Tài Xī (KI-3) on both sides of the body.

6. We know from a more explicit version in the *Líng Shū* that this does not mean to insert one needle on each side (to a total of three needles), but to insert one needle in the center and one to its side.

I.30 On Pricking the Yīn and Yáng Channels of the Hands and Feet*
Shǒu zú yīn yáng jīng mài cì lùn
手足陰陽經脈刺論

Note:

* Excerpted from *Líng Shū* 12, *Jīng shuǐ* 經水 (Channels and Waterways).

Line 1

(一)岐伯曰：足陽明，五臟六腑之海也 。(二)其脈大血多 。(三)氣盛壯熱，刺此者，不深不散，不留不瀉也 。

(1) Qíbó said: "The foot yángmíng [vessel] is the sea of the five viscera and six bowels. (2) Its vessel is large and its blood profuse. (3) In patients with exuberant qì and vigorous heat [effusion], when pricking this vessel, do not prick deeply, do not dissipate, do not retain [the needle], and do not drain.

Line 2

(一)足陽明刺深六分，留十呼 。(二)足太陽深五分，留七呼 。(三)足少陽深四分，留五呼 。(四)足少陰深三分，留四呼 。(五)足太陰深二分，留三呼 。(六)足厥陰，深一分，留二呼 。

(1) On the foot yángmíng [vessel], prick to a depth of six *fēn* and retain [the needle] for ten breaths. (2) On the foot tàiyáng [vessel, prick] to a depth of five *fēn* and retain [the needle] for seven breaths. (3) On the foot shàoyáng [vessel, prick] to a depth of four *fēn* and retain [the needle] for five breaths. (4) On the foot shàoyīn [vessel, prick] to a depth of three *fēn* and retain [the needle] for four breaths. (5) On the foot tàiyīn [vessel, prick] to a depth of two *fēn* and retain [the needle] for three breaths. (6) On the foot juéyīn [vessel, prick] to a depth of one *fēn* and retain [the needle] for two breaths.

Line 3

(一)手之陰陽，其受氣之道近，其氣之來疾 。(二)其刺深者，皆無過二分，其留，皆無過一呼 。(三)刺而過此者，則脫氣 。

(1) In the yīn and yáng [vessels] of the hand, the path by which they receive qì [from the lung] is close-by, and the arrival of qì is quick.* (2) When pricking [these vessels], the depth should never exceed two *fēn* and [the needle] should never be retained for longer than one breath. (3) If you exceed these limits when pricking [the hand yīn and yáng vessels], qì desertion will result."

Note:

   * Because the hands are closer to the lung than the legs, the distance that qì has to travel to reach the endpoint of these vessels is shorter.

I.31 On the Tip and Root[*]
Biāo běn lùn
標本論

Note:

* Excerpted from *Sù Wèn* 65, *Biāo běn bìng chuán lùn* 標本病傳論 (On the Tip and Root and on Disease Transmission).

Line 1

(一)岐伯曰：先病而後逆者，治其本；先逆而後病者，治其本 。(二)先寒而後生病者，治其本；先病而後生寒者，治其本 。(三)先熱而後生病者，治其本 。(四)先泄而後生他病者，治其本 。(五)必且調之，乃治其他病 。(六)先病而後中滿者，治其標 。(七)先病而後泄者治其本 。(八)先中滿而後煩心者，治其本 。

(1) Qíbó said: "When illness precedes counterflow, treat the root. When counterflow precedes illness, treat the root. (2) When cold precedes the formation of illness, treat the root. When illness precedes the formation of cold, treat the root. (3) When heat precedes the formation of illness, treat the root. (4) When diarrhea appears first before the formation of other illness, treat the root. (5) You must first regulate this [condition] before treating the other illnesses. (6) When illness appears first before fullness in the center, treat the tip. (7) When illness appears first before diarrhea, treat the root. (8) When fullness in the center appears first before vexation in the heart, treat the root.

Line 2

(一)有客氣有同氣，大小便不利，治其標 。大小便利，治其本 。(二)病發而
有餘，本而標之 。先治其本，後治其標 。(三)病發而不足，標而本之 。先治
其標，後治其本 。

(1) [Regardless of the presence of] guest qì or shared qì [as the root condition],*
when defecation and urination are inhibited [as the tip symptom], treat the tip.
When defecation and urination are not inhibited, treat the root. (2) When illness
arises in conjunction with [signs of] excess [of evil qì], [apply the principle of] "the
root [first] and then the tip." First treat the root and then treat the tip. (3) When illness arises in conjunction with [signs of insufficiency], [apply the principle of] "the
tip first and then the root." First treat the tip and then treat the root.

Note:

    * My translation of this phrase follows the commentary tradition of the *Sù Wèn* source.
"Guest qì" refers to evil qì intruding from the outside, while "shared qì" is the body's right
qì.

Line 3

(一)謹詳察間甚，以意調之 。間者併行 ；甚為獨行 。(二)先大小便不利而
後生他病者，治其本也 。

(1) Carefully examine the degree of severity in detail and then apply your intention
to regulate the condition. In mild cases, address both [the root and tip at the same
time]; in severe cases, address only one. (2) If inhibited defecation and urination
precede the formation of other illness, treat the root."

160

I.32 Pricking Nobles and Commoners
Cì wáng gōng bù yī
刺王公布衣

Line 1

岐伯曰：膏粱藿菽之味，何可同也 。

Qíbó said: "How could [the treatment of disease] be identical [in patients who eat] rich and fancy foods and [in those who eat] beans and vegetables?*

Note:

> * I.e., upper-class patients who live sheltered lives in physical comfort and consume an abundance of rich foods, in contrast to the common people who work hard, live in poor conditions, and are under-nourished.

Line 2

(一)氣滑則出疾；氣濇則出遲 。(二)氣悍則針小而入淺；氣濇則針大而入深 。(三)深則欲留；淺則欲疾 。(四)以此觀之，刺布衣者，深而留之；刺大人者，微以徐之 。(五)此皆因其慓悍滑利也 。(六)寒痹內熱，刺布衣以火焠之；刺大人，以藥熨之 。

(1) When the flow of qì is smooth, remove [the needle] quickly. When the flow of qì is halting, remove [the needle] slowly. (2) When the flow of qì is fierce, use small needles and insert them shallowly. When the flow of qì is halting, use big needles and insert them deeply. (3) When [pricking] deeply, you want to retain [the needles]. When [pricking] shallowly, you want to act quickly. (4) If you observe these guidelines, when pricking commoners, [prick] deeply and retain [the needles]; when pricking important people, use small [needles] and treat [the patient] in a dignified fashion. (5) The reason for this is that [the flow of their qì] is fierce, smooth, and uninhibited. (6) In the treatment of cold impediment with internal heat, when pricking commoners, use fire and red-hot pricking; when pricking important people, use medicinals and apply them in hot compresses."

I.33 Pricking Normal People, Black and White, Fat and Thin*
Cì cháng rén hēi bái féi shòu
刺常人黑白肥瘦

Note:

* Excerpted from *Líng Shū* 38, *Nì shùn féi shòu* 逆順肥瘦 (Treating the Fat and Thin According to Circumstance).

Line 1

(一)岐伯曰：年質壯大，血氣充盈，膚革堅固。(二)因加以邪，刺此者，深而留，此肥人也。

(1) Qíbó said: "In strong adults in their prime, the qì and blood are abundant and the skin is firm. (2) Therefore, when you prick this type of patients after they have contracted [external] evil, prick deeply and retain [the needle]. This is [the method for] fat people.

Line 2

(一)廣肩腋項、肉厚、皮黑色、唇臨臨然，其血黑以濁，其氣濇以遲。(二)其為人也，貪於取與。(三)刺此者，深而留之，多益其數也。

(1) In people with broad shoulders and necks, thick flesh, blackish skin,* and full lips, their blood is black and turbid; their qì is halting and slow. (2) It is the nature of such people to covet taking things from others. (3) When you prick this type of patients, prick deeply and retain [the needle]. Also, increase the number of prickings by a lot.

Note:

> * The terms "black" and "white" here obviously do not refer to people of African and European descent respectively, but rather to people with darker and paler complexion, regardless of their racial heritage.

Line 3

(一)瘦人，皮薄色白、肉廉廉然、薄脣、輕言，其血氣清，易脫於氣，易損於血 。(二)刺此者，淺而疾之 。

(1) In thin people with fine skin and a pale complexion, emaciated flesh, thin lips and quiet speech, the blood and qì are clear and they have a tendency to suffer from desertion of qì and detriment to the blood. (2) When pricking this type of patients, prick shallowly and quickly.

Line 4

(一)刺肥人者，以秋冬之齊 。(二)刺瘦人者，以春夏之齊 。

(1) When pricking fat patients, treat them all in the fall and winter. (2) When pricking thin patients, treat them all in the spring and summer."

I.34 Pricking Strong Persons[1,2]
Cì zhuàng shì
刺壯士

Notes:

1. Literally meaning "warrior" or "hero," the closest modern equivalent would probably be "athlete," in other words, people with physiques characterized by great physical strength.

2. Excerpted from *Líng Shū* 38, *Nì shùn féi shòu* 逆順肥瘦 (Treating the Fat and Thin According to Circumstance).

Line 1

岐伯曰：壯士真骨、堅肉、緩節 。

Qíbó said: "Strong persons have solid bones, firm flesh, and loose joints.

Line 2

(一)此人重，則氣濇血濁 。(二)刺此者，深而留之，多益其數 。(三)勁則氣滑血清 。(四)刺此者，淺而疾之 。

(1) If such a person is heavy,* their qì is halting and their blood turbid. (2) When pricking this kind of person, prick deeply and retain [the needle]. Also increase the number of prickings by a lot. (3) If such a person is full of vigor, their qì is smooth and clear. (4) When pricking this kind of person, prick shallowly and quickly."

Note:

* In the context of this line, "heavy" (and "full of vigor" in the following line) describes both the body and the personality, in the sense of lethargic or passive.

I.35 Pricking Infants[*]
Cì yīng ér
刺嬰兒

Note:

[*] Excerpted from *Líng Shū* 38, *Nì shùn féi shòu* 逆順肥瘦 (Treating the Fat and Thin According to Circumstance).

(一)岐伯曰：嬰兒者，其肉脆，血少氣弱 。(二)刺此者，以毫針，淺刺而疾發針，日再刺可也 。

(1) Qíbó said: "Infants have brittle flesh, scant blood, and weak qì. (2) When pricking them, use fine needles, prick shallowly, and quickly remove the needle. You may prick twice in one day."

I.36 Differences in Pricking a Person's Left and Right Side, Upper Part and Lower Part, Vacuity and Repletion*
Rén shēn zuǒ yòu shàng xià xū shí bù tóng cì
人身左右上下虛實不同刺

Note:

> * Excerpted from *Sù Wèn* 5, *Yīn yáng yīng xiáng dà lùn* 陰陽應像大論 (Great Treatise on the Correspondences and Manifestations of Yīn and Yáng).

Line 1

(一)岐伯曰：天不足西北，故西北方陰也，而人右耳目不如左明也 。(二)地不滿東南，故東南方陽也，而人左手足不如右強也 。(三)東方陽也 。陽者其精并於上，并於上，則上明而下虛，故使耳目聰明，而手足不便 。(四)西方陰也 。陰者其精并於下，并於下，則下盛而上虛，故使耳目不聰明，而手足便也 。

(1) Qíbó said: "Heaven is insufficient in the Northwest. Therefore, the direction of northwest is [associated with] yīn, and a person's right ears and eyes are not as bright* as those on the left side. (2) The earth is not full in the Southeast. Therefore, the direction of southeast is [associated with] yáng, and a person's left hands and feet are not as strong as those on the right side. (3) The eastern direction is yáng. The essence of yáng is associated with above. Since [the East] is associated with above, the upper part [of human bodies in the East] is bright and the lower part is vacuous. Therefore the ears and eyes are perceptive, but the hands and feet do not function smoothly. (4) The western direction is yīn. The essence of yīn is associated with below. Since [the west] is associated with below, the lower part [of human bodies in the West] is exuberant and the upper part is vacuous. Therefore the ears and eyes are not perceptive, but the hands and feet function smoothly.

Note:

> * Here in the sense of "perceptive."

Line 2

(一)故俱感於邪，其在上則右甚，在下則左甚 。(二)此天地陰陽所不能移也，故邪居之 。(三)蓋天有精，地有形，天有八紀，地有五理，故能為萬物之父母 。(四)清陽上天，濁陰歸地 。是故天地之動靜，神明之綱紀，故能以生長收藏，終而復始 。(五)惟賢人上配天以養頭，下象地以養足，中傍人事以養五臟 。

(1) For this reason, whenever a person has contracted an [external] evil, if it is in the upper body, it will be worse on the right; if it is in the lower body, it will be worse on the left. (2) The reason for this is that heaven and earth, yīn and yáng have aspects that they are unable to alter,[1] and evil is therefore able to take up residence there. (3) Now, heaven has essence and earth has form. In heaven, there are eight guiding principles;[2] on earth, there are five patterns.[3] For this reason, they are able to be father and mother to the myriad things. (4) Clear yáng rises up to heaven, turbid yīn returns to earth. For this reason, the movement and stillness of heaven and earth and the guiding principle of the spirit light are able to end and begin anew [in the transformations of] generation, growth, gathering, and storing. (5) It is only the sage who is able to match heaven above to nourish the head, resemble earth below to nourish the feet, and in the middle partake of human affairs to nourish the five viscera.

Notes:

1. Instead of *yí* 移, the parallel phrase in the *Sù Wèn* has *quán* 全, "to complete."
2. *Jì* 紀 literally means "main thread" and from there by extension "organizing principle" or "time marker." Here, the commentary to the *Sù Wèn* explains it as a reference to the eight seasonal time markers of the year, i.e., the beginnings of the four seasons, the spring and fall equinox, and the summer and winter solstice.
3. According to the *Sù Wèn* commentary, "five patterns" refers to the five directions, east, south, north, west, and the center.

Line 3

(一)天氣通於肺，地氣通於嗌，風氣通於肝，雷氣通於心，谷氣通於脾，雨氣通於腎。(二)六經為川，腸胃為海，九竅為水注之器。(三)以天地為之陰陽，陽之汗，以天地之雨名之；陽之氣，以天地之疾風名之。(四)暴風象雷，逆風象陽。(五)故治不法天之紀，不用地之理，則災害至矣！(六)故邪風之至，疾如風雨。

(1) The qì of heaven flows through the lung; the qì of earth flows through the throat; the qì of wind flows through the liver; the qì of thunder flows through the heart; the qì of valleys flows through the spleen; the qì of rain flows through the kidney. (2) The six channels constitute rivers, the intestine and stomach constitute seas, and the nine orifices constitute vessels for pouring water. (3) Taking heaven and earth as [corresponding to] yīn and yáng [in the human body], the sweat of [effusing] yáng [in the human body] is described by rain in heaven and earth; the qì of yáng [in the human body] is described by the gales in heaven and earth.[1] (4) Fulminant wind resembles thunder, counterflow wind resembles yáng [fire flaming upward].[2] (5) For this reason, if in your treatments you fail to follow heaven's guiding principles and to use earth's patterns, disaster will ensue. (6) Therefore the arrival of evil wind will be swift like wind and rain.

Notes:

1. In this line, "heaven and earth" has the sense of "natural environment."
2. The parallel phrase in the *Sù Wèn* has qì 氣 here instead of *fēng* 風.

Line 4

(一)故善治者治皮毛；其次治肌膚；其次治筋脈；其次治六腑；其次治五臟。(二)治五臟者，半死半生也。(三)故天之邪氣，感則害人五臟；水穀之寒熱，感則害人六腑；地之濕氣，感則害人皮膚筋脈。(四)故善用針者，從陰引陽，從陽引陰；以右治左，以左治右；以我知彼，以表知裏；以觀過與不及之理，見微則過，用之不殆。

(1) Therefore, a person skilled in treating [disease] treats [disease while it only affects the superficial layer of] the body hair. Next [in skill], a person treats the flesh and skin.[1] Next, a person treats the sinews and vessels. Next, a person treats the six bowels. Next, a person treats the five viscera.[2] (2) When you treat [disease only after it has already affected] the five viscera, [the patient] has half a chance of dying and

168

half a chance of surviving. (3) For this reason, contracting the evil qì of heaven will injure the person's five viscera. Contracting cold or heat from water and grain will injure the person's six bowels. Contracting the damp qì of earth will injure the person's skin, joints, and vessels. (4) For this reason, a person skilled at using needles draws [a disease] from yīn out through yáng, draws [a disease] from yáng out through yīn; uses the right [half of the body] to treat the left, uses the left [half of the body] to treat the right; uses [his or her own body] to know [the body of others]; uses the exterior to know the interior; and uses the observation of the patterns of excess and insufficiency to see the slight [abnormality] that will result in excess.[3] Using these [principles], there is no danger.

Notes:

1. The parallel phrase in the *Sù Wèn* has *jī ròu* 肌肉 "flesh" here instead of *jī fū* 肌膚 ("flesh and skin").
2. This line expresses the same notion as the better-known ideal to "treat disease before it arises" (*zhì wèi bìng* 治未病).
3. I.e. is able to recognize illness based on minute changes in the body before it results in dangerous excess.

II. The Root Meaning of the Classic of Difficulties
Nàn jīng běn yì
難經本意

II.1 The First Difficulty
Yī nàn
一難

Line 1

十二經皆有動脈，獨取寸口，以決五臟六腑，死生吉凶之法，何謂也？

"The pulse moves[1] in all twelve channels. What does it mean that we only choose *cùn kǒu*[2] in the method for determining life and death and auspicious and inauspicious states in the five viscera and six bowels?"

Notes:

1. In the following lines, the term *dòng* 動, here translated literally as "to move," describes the movement of qì in the vessels, as it can be detected by pulse diagnosis, so it could also be translated less literally below as "is detectable as pulse."
2. Lit. "inch opening."

Line 2

(一)十二經皆有動脈者 。(二)如手太陰脈：動中府 、雲門 、天府 、俠白 。(三)手陽明脈：動合谷 、陽谿 。(四)手少陰脈：動極泉 。(五)手太陽脈：動天窗 。(六)手厥陰脈：動勞宮 。(七)手少陽脈：動禾髎 。(八)足太陰脈：動箕門 、衝門 。(九)足陽明脈：動衝陽 、大迎 、人迎 、氣衝 。(十)足少陰脈：動太溪 、陰谷 。(十一)足太陽脈：動委中 。(十二)足厥陰脈：動太衝 、五里 、陰廉 。(十三)足少陽脈：動下關 、聽會之類也 。

(1) "The twelve channels all have [locations where] the pulse moves. (2) For example, the hand tàiyīn vessel moves at Zhōng Fǔ (LU-1), Yún Mén (LU-2), Tiān Fǔ (LU-3), and Xiá Bái (LU-4). (3) The hand yángmíng vessel moves at Hé Gǔ (LI-4) and Yáng Xī (LI-5). (4) The hand shàoyīn vessel moves at Jí Quán (HT-1). (5) The hand tàiyáng vessel moves at Tiān Chuāng (SI-16). (6) The hand juéyīn vessel moves at Láo Gōng (PC-8). (7) The hand shàoyáng vessel moves at Hé Liáo (TB-22). (8) The foot tàiyīn vessel moves at Jī Mén (SP-11). (9) The foot yángmíng vessel moves at Chōng Yáng (ST-42), Dà Yíng (ST-5), Rén Yíng (ST-9), and Qì Chōng (ST-30). (10) The foot shàoyīn vessel moves at Tài Xī (KI-3) and Yīn Gǔ (KI-10). (11) The foot tàiyáng vessel moves at Wěi Zhōng (BL-40). (12) The foot juéyīn vessel moves at Tài Chōng (LV-3), Wǔ Lǐ*, and Yīn Lián (LV-11). (13) The foot shàoyáng vessel moves at Xià Guān (ST-7) and Tīng Huì (GB-2).

Note:

* This point is identified with Láo Gōng 勞宮 (PC-8).

Line 3

(一)謂之經者, 以榮衛之流行, 經常不息者而言。(二)謂之脈者, 以血理之分衺行體者而言也。(三)故經者徑也。脈者陌也。越人之意。(四)蓋謂凡此十二經, 經皆有動脈, 如上文所云者。

(1) What we call 'channels' refers to the flow of construction and defense [qì], which is constant and unceasing. (2) What we call 'vessels' refers to the divisions in the blood patterns that run lengthwise in the body. (3) For this reason, the channels are throughways and the vessels are paths between fields. This is what the person from Yuè* meant. (4) Now, when we refer to all these twelve channels, each of the channels has moving vessels, as stated in the above lines.

Note:

* I.e., Biǎn Què 扁鵲, the author of the Nàn Jīng.

Line 4

今置不取，又獨取寸口，以決臟腑死生吉凶，何耶！

Not to select the locations [mentioned] here, but only to select *cùn kǒu* in order to determine the [state of the] viscera and bowels, life and death, good luck or misfortune, why would that be!

Line 5

(一)然：寸口者，脈之大會，手太陰之脈動也 。(二)寸口，謂氣口也。居手太陰魚際卻行一寸之分 。(三)氣口之下曰關，曰尺 。

(1) Answer: *cùn kǒu* is the great meeting point of the vessels and [reveals] the movement of the hand tàiyīn vessel. (2) *Cùn kǒu* refers to *qì kǒu*.[1] It is located on the hand tàiyīn [vessel], separated from the thenar eminence by one *cùn*. (3) Below *qì kǒu* is called *guān* and [below *guān*] is called *chǐ*.[2]

Notes:

1. Lit. the opening of qì.
2. I.e., the locations for taking the bar (*guān* 關) and cubit (*chǐ* 尺) pulses, respectively.

Line 6

(一)云者，而榮衛之行於陽者，二十五度，行於陰者，亦二十五度 。(二)出入陰陽，參交互注，無少間斷，五十度畢 。(三)適當漏下百刻，為一晬時，又明日之平旦矣，迺復會於手太陰 。(四)此寸口所以為五臟六腑之所始終，而法有取於是焉 。

(1) It is said that the movement of construction and defense [qì] in yáng is 25 measures, the movement in yīn is also 25 measures. (2) [The contents of the channels] exit and enter yīn and yáng, intermingle and pour into each other, never stopping even for a moment, completing [their cycle] in 50 measures. (3) Arriving at the time it takes a water clock to drip down a hundred markings, this constitutes one full cycle, as well as the dawn of the new day, upon which they again meet in the hand tàiyīn [vessel]. (4) This is the reason why *cùn kǒu* is the beginning and end of [the

movement of qì through] the five viscera and six bowels and why a method exists for taking this [point to examine the flow of qì in all the vessels].

Line 7

(一)人一呼一吸為一息，每刻一百三十五息，每時八刻，計一千八十息。(二)十二時九十六刻，計一萬二千九百六十息，刻之餘分，得五百四十息，合一萬三千五百息也。(三)一息脈行六寸，每二刻二百七十息，脈行一十六丈二尺。(四)每時八刻，脈行六十四丈八尺。

(1) In humans, one breath consists of one inhalation and one exhalation. Every marking [of the water clock] is [the equivalent of] 135 breaths, and every hour contains eight markings, which adds up to 1080 breaths. (2) Twelve hours mean 96 markings, which adds up to 12,960 breaths. The remaining markings takes 540 breaths, which brings the total to 13,500 breaths. (3) In one breath, the [contents of the] vessels travel 6 *cùn*. Every two markings take 270 breaths, during which time the [contents of the] vessels travel 16 *zhàng* and two *chǐ*. (4) In every hour, or eight markings, the [contents of the] vessels travel 64 *zhàng* and 8 *chǐ*.

Line 8

(一)榮衛四周於身，十二時計九十六刻，脈行七百七十七丈六尺，為四十八周身。(二)刻之餘分，行二周身，得三十二丈四尺，總之為五十度周身，脈得八百一十丈也。(三)此呼吸之息，脈行之數，周身之度，合晝夜百刻之詳也。(四)行陽行陰，謂行晝行夜。

(1) Construction and defense qì cycle through the body four times, which takes twelve hours or a total of 96 markings, during which the [contents of the] vessels travel 777 *zhàng* and six *chǐ*, which means 48 cycles through the body. (2) For the remaining markings, [the vessel contents] travel through the body in two cycles, reaching 32 *zhàng* and 4 *chǐ*. This makes a total of 50 times of traveling through the body, during which the [contents of the] vessels reach 810 *zhàng*. (3) These are the details of breathing with inhalations and exhalations, of the distance traveled by the [contents of the] vessels, of the times of cycles through the body, and of a total of 100 markings in one day and night. (4) Traveling through yáng and traveling through yīn refers to traveling through the day and traveling through the night."

II.2 The Seventh Difficulty
Qī nàn
七難

Line 1

(一)經言少陽之至，乍大乍小，乍短乍長；陽明之至，浮大而短；太陽之至，洪大而長；太陰之至，緊大而長；少陰之至，緊細而微；厥陰之至，沉短而數 。(二)此六者，是平脈邪，將病脈邪？

(1) The classic says: "The arrival of the shàoyáng pulse is now large now small, now short now long. The arrival of the yángmíng pulse is floating, large, and short. The arrival of the tàiyáng pulse is surging, large, and long. The arrival of the tàiyīn pulse is tight, large, and long. The arrival of the shàoyīn pulse is tight, fine, and slight. The arrival of the juéyīn pulse is sunken, short, and rapid. (2) Are these six types normal pulses or pathologic pulses?"

Line 2

(一)然：皆王¹脈也 。(二)六脈者之王，說見下文 。

(1) Answer: "They are all the pulses of the ruling qì.² (2) For an explanation of the ruling [qì] of the six pulses, see the following lines."

Notes:

1. The character *wáng* 王 could also be read as *wàng* 旺 in the sense of "pulses of [seasonal] effulgence]. I read the character literally as "act in the role of the king," i.e. "rule."
2. In other words, these pulse characteristics indicate neither a normal (i.e., healthy) nor an abnormal state of qì in the body, but reflect the changes of qì in the seasonal cycle. This chapter hence shows the importance of always reading a patient's body as part of the larger cosmological changes in the universe instead of as an isolated individual.

Line 3

其氣以何月各王幾日？

"In which month and for how many days does each qì rule?"

Line 4

（一）然：冬至之後，得甲子少陽王，復得甲子陽明王，復得甲子太陽王，
復得甲子太陰王，復得甲子少陰王，復得甲子厥陰王。（二）王各六十日，六
六，三百六十日，以成一歲。此三陽、三陰之王時日大要也。（三）上文言三
陽、三陰之王脈，此言三陽、三陰之王時，當其時，則見其脈也。

(1) **Answer:** "After the winter solstice, shàoyáng rules for the first *jiǎ zǐ** cycle; for the next *jiǎ zǐ* cycle, yángmíng rules; for the next *jiǎ zǐ* cycle, tàiyáng rules; for the next *jiǎ zǐ* cycle, tàiyīn rules; for the next *jiǎ zǐ* cycle, shàoyīn rules; for the next *jiǎ zǐ* cycle, juéyīn rules. (2) Each rules for sixty days, to a total of six [*jiā* cycles] times six or 360 days, which completes one year. This is the general principle on the ruling seasons and days of the three yáng and three yīn. (3) When the above text speaks of the ruling pulses of the three yīn and three yáng, it refers to the times when the three yáng and three yīn [qì] rule. Matching their times, you can then see their pulse.

Note:

> * *Jiǎ zǐ* 甲子 refers to the first of the ten heavenly stems and of the twelve earthly branches respectively. Here, it stands for one complete cycle of 60 days each. The stems and branches (*gān zhī* 干支) system is used in the traditional Chinese calendar to count cycles of 60, both in regard to years and days.

Line 5

劉溫曰：至真要論云：厥陰之至，其脈弦；少陰之至，其脈鈎；太陰之至，其脈沉；少陽之至，大而浮；陽明之至，短而濇；太陽之至，大而長。

Liú Wēn quotes the *'Great Treatise on the Essentials of Supreme Truth'*: 'When juéyīn arrives, its pulse is stringlike. When shàoyīn arrives, its pulse is like a hook. When tàiyīn arrives, its pulse is sunken. When shàoyáng arrives, [its pulse is] large and floating. When yángmíng arrives, [its pulse is] short and rough. When tàiyáng arrives, [its pulse is] large and long.'

Note:

　　* I.e., *Sù Wèn*, chapter 74.

Line 6

(一)亦隨天地之氣卷舒也。如春弦、夏洪、秋毛、冬石之類。(二)則五運六氣四時，亦皆應之而見於脈耳。

(1) Moreover, [the pulses] furl and unfurl in accordance with the qì of heaven and earth, for example being stringlike in spring, surging in summer, downy in the fall, and stone-like in the winter. (2) Thus, when looking at the pulse, you always have to [read it] also as responding to the five movements, six qì, and four seasons.

Line 7

(一)若平人氣象論，太陽脈至洪大而長，少陽脈至乍數乍疏乍短乍長，陽明脈至浮大而短。(二)難經引之，以論三陰三陽之脈者，以陰陽始生之淺深而言之也。

(1) As the chapter 'On the Manifestations of Qì in Healthy Persons' states, 'when the tàiyáng pulse arrives, it is surging, large, and long; when the shàoyáng pulse arrives, it is now rapid now sparse, now short now long; when the yángmíng pulse arrives, it is floating, large, and short.' (2) The *Nàn Jīng* quotes these to discuss the three yīn and three yáng pulses, to speak of them in terms of the shallowness and depth of the origin of yīn and yáng."

Note:

* I.e., *Sù Wèn*, chapter 18.

II.3 The Twelfth Difficulty
Shí èr nàn
十二難

Line 1

(一)經言五臟脈已絕於內，用針者反實其外；五臟脈已絕於外，用針者反實其內 。(二)內外之絕，何以別之？

(1) The classic states: "If the pulses of the five viscera are expired on the inside, in applying needles it is wrong to fill the outside. If the pulses of the five viscera are expired on the outside in applying needles, it is wrong to fill the inside." (2) "How do you distinguish between expiry on the inside and expiry on the outside?"

Line 2

(一)然：五臟脈已絕於內者，腎肝氣已絕於內也，而醫反補其心肺 。(二)五臟脈已絕於外者，其心肺脈已絕於外也，而醫反補其腎肝 。(三)陽絕補陰，陰絕補陽，是謂實實虛虛，損不足而益有餘 。(四)如此死者，醫殺之耳 。

(1) Answer: "If the pulses of the five viscera are expired on the inside, it means that the qì of the kidney and liver is expired on the inside, and a physician would be mistaken to supplement the patient's heart and lung. (2) If the pulses of the five viscera are expired on the outside, it means that the pulses of the heart and lung are expired on the outside, and a physician would be mistaken to supplement the kidney and liver. (3) To supplement yīn when yáng is expired, or to supplement yáng when yīn is expired, this is what is meant by 'making repletion [more] replete and making vacuity [more] vacuous, reducing insufficiency and increasing superabundance.' (4) If a patient dies under these conditions, it is the physician who has killed them!

Line 3

(一)靈樞云：凡將用針，必先診脈，視氣之劇易，乃可以治也 。(二)又云：
所謂五臟之氣已絕於內者，脈口氣內絕不至 。反取其外之病處與陽經之合，
有留針以致陽氣，陽氣至則內重竭。(三)重竭，則死 。其死也無氣以動，故
靜 。(四)所謂五臟之氣已絕於外者，脈口氣外絕不至 。反取其四末之輸，有
留針以致其陰氣，陰氣至則陽氣反入 。(五)入則逆，逆則死矣 。其死也陰氣
有餘，故躁 。(六)此靈樞以脈口內外言陰陽也 。(七)越人以心肺腎肝內外別
陰陽，其理亦由是也 。

(1) The *Líng Shū* states: 'Whenever you apply needles, you must first examine the pulse and observe the severity or ease of the qì. Only afterwards can you apply [needles] to treat the patient.' (2) It also states: 'What is meant by expiry of the qì of the five viscera on the inside is that the qì in the openings of the vessels is expired on the inside and hence fails to arrive. If you wrongly select a disease location on the outside or a uniting point* of the yáng vessels [as points to needle], and leave the needles in to make the patient's yáng qì arrive, when the yáng qì arrives, it results in doubling the exhaustion on the inside. (3) Doubling the exhaustion results in death. In this case, the death [is due to] an absence of qì to make any movement, and hence [it is marked by] stillness. (4) What is meant by expiry of the qì of the five viscera on the outside is that the qì in the openings of the vessels is expired on the outside and hence fails to arrive. If you wrongly select the transport points on the four extremities and leave the needles in to make the patient's yīn qì arrive, when the yīn qì arrives, it results in yáng qì wrongly entering [the yīn half of the body instead]. (5) [Yáng qì] entering [the inside of the body] results in counterflow, and counterflow results in death. In this case, the death [is due to] an overabundance of yīn qì, and hence [it is marked by] agitation.' (6) In this quotation, the *Líng Shū* uses the inside and outside vessel openings to speak of yīn and yáng. (7) The person from Yuè uses the outside of the heart and lung and the inside of the kidney and liver to distinguish between yīn and yáng. Its underlying principle is also rooted in this."

Note:

   * A reference to the *hé xuè* 合穴, "uniting points" (i.e., transport points) of the major channels.

II.4 The Twenty-Second Difficulty
Èr shí èr nàn
二十二難

Line 1

經言脈有是動，有所生病，一脈變為二病者，何也？

"What does it mean when the classic says: 'The pulse can be marked by stirring and it can be marked by illness forming'? How can a single pulse change in response to two illnesses?"

Note:

* I.e., illnesses of the qì and illnesses of the blood.

Line 2

(一)然：經言是動者，氣也 。(二)所生病者，血也 。(三)邪在氣，氣為是動；邪在血，血為所生病. (四)氣主呴*之，血主濡之 。(五)氣留而不行者，為氣先病也；血壅而不濡者，為血後病也 。(六)故先為是動，後所生也 。

(1) Answer: "When the classic speaks of stirring, it refers to the qì. (2) When it speaks of illness forming, it refers to the blood. (3) If the evil is in the qì, the qì will stir because of it. If the evil is in the blood, the blood will form illness because of it. (4) The qì is in charge of warming the body; the blood is in charge of moistening it. (5) When qì lodges and fails to move, it first causes disease in the qì. When blood becomes congested and fails to moisten, it afterwards causes disease in the blood. (6) Therefore, [evil] first causes stirring and afterwards forms illness."

Note:

* My translation is based on the commentary tradition to the *Nàn Jīng. Xǔ* 呴 literally means "to breathe on," hence the sense here of qì warming the body by blowing through it like a warm breeze.

179

II.5 The Thirty-Fifth Difficulty
Sān shí wǔ nàn
三十五難

Line 1

五臟各有所腑皆相近，而心、肺獨去大腸、小腸遠者，何也？

"Each of the five viscera has a specific bowel [associated with it], which in each case is located nearby. And yet, only the heart and lung are far removed from the large and small intestine. Why is that?"

Line 2

(一)然：經言心榮肺衛，通行陽氣，故居在上。(二)大腸、小腸，傳陰氣而下，故居在下，所以相去而遠也。

(1) Answer: "The classic says that the heart is [in charge of] construction and the lung is [in charge of] defense. They provide for the free flow of yáng qì and therefore reside in the upper body. (2) The large and small intestine convey yīn qì downward and therefore reside in the lower body. For this reason, they are far away from each other."

II.6 The Fortieth Difficulty
Sì shí nàn
四十難

Line 1

(一)經言肝主色，心主臭，脾主味，肺主聲，腎主液。(二)鼻者肺之候，而反知香臭。(三)耳者腎之候，而反聞聲。(四)其義何也？

(1) "The classic says that the liver governs colors, the heart governs smells, the spleen governs tastes, the lung governs sounds, and the kidney governs fluids. (2) The nose is the indicator of the lung, and yet it conversely knows [the difference between] fragrance and stench. (3) The ears are the indicator of the kidney and yet they conversely hear sounds. (4) What is the meaning of this?"

Line 2

(一)然：肺者西方金也。金生於巳；巳者南方火；火者心。(二)心主臭，故令鼻知香臭。(三)腎者北方水也。(四)水生於申；申者西方金；金者肺。(五)肺主聲，故令耳聞聲。

(1) Answer: "The lung is [associated with] the western direction and with metal. Metal is engendered in *sì*.[1] *Sì* is [associated with] the southern direction and with fire. Fire is [associated with] the heart. (2) The heart governs smells and hence allows the nose to know [the difference between] fragrance and stench. (3) The kidney is [associated with] the northern direction and with water. (4) Water is engendered in *shēn*.[2] *Shēn* is [associated with] the western direction and with metal. (5) Metal is [associated with] the lung. The lung governs sounds and hence allows the ears to hear sounds.

Notes:

1. The sixth of the twelve earthly branches (*dì zhī* 地支).
2. The ninth of the twelve earthly branches.

Line 3

(一)四明陳氏曰：臭者心所主，鼻者肺之竅，心之脈上肺，故令鼻能知香臭也。(二)聲者肺所主，耳者腎之竅，腎之脈上肺，故令耳能聞聲也。(三)愚按越人此說，蓋以五行相生之義而言，且見其相因而為用也。

(1) Chén Sì-míng states: '[The sense of] smell is governed by the heart, but the nose is the orifice of the lung. The heart vessel ascends to the lung and therefore allows the nose to be able to know fragrance and stench. (2) [The sense of] hearing is governed by the lung, but the ears are the orifices of the kidney. The kidney vessel ascends to the lung and therefore allows the ears to be able to hear sounds.' (3) In accordance with the present explanation by the person from Yuè, I have discussed this issue in terms of the meaning of the theory of mutual generation among the five phases, seeing their mutual causation [in each other] and applying that."

II.7 The Forty-Third Difficulty
Sì shí sān nàn
四十三難

Line 1

人不食飲，七日而死者，何也？

"Why is it that if people don't eat or drink, they die after seven days?"

Line 2

(一)然：人胃中，常有留穀二斗，水一斗五升，故平人日再至圊，一行二升半，日中五升，七日五七三斗五升，而水穀盡矣。(二)故平人不食飲，七日而死者，水穀津液俱盡，即死矣。(三)水去則榮散。(四)穀消則衛亡。榮散衛亡，神無所依，故死。

(1) Answer: "Inside a person's stomach, we commonly find a reserve of 2 *dǒu* of solids and 1 *dǒu* and 5 *shēng* of liquids.* For this reason, a healthy person, who has two bowel movements per day [and eliminates] 2.5 *shēng* in one movement, thus 5 *shēng* in one day, eliminates 5 times 7 *shēng*, or 3 *dǒu* and 5 *shēng*, in seven days, after which all solids and liquids will be used up. (2) Therefore, the reason why a healthy person who does not eat or drink will die in seven days is that all the solids and liquids [in their stomach] will be used up then, resulting in death. (3) When the liquids are gone, construction [*qì*] dissipates. (4) When the solids are dispersed, defense [*qì*] perishes. When construction is dissipated and defense perished, the spirit has no support, which causes death."

Note:

* "Water" and "grain" are standard terms for the solid and liquid parts of our diet.

II.8 The Forty-Sixth Difficulty
Sì shí liù nàn
四十六難

Line 1

老人臥而不寐，少壯寐而不寤者，何也？

"Why is it that old people rest without sleeping while strong youngsters sleep without waking up?"

Line 2

(一)然：經言少壯者血氣盛，肌肉滑，氣道通，榮衛之行不失於常。(二)故晝日精，夜不寤也。(三)老人血氣衰，肌肉不滑，榮衛之道濇。(四)故晝日不能精，夜不得寐也。(五)老臥不寐，少寐不寤係乎榮衛血氣之有餘不足也。

(1) Answer: "According to the classic, in strong youngsters blood and qì are exuberant, the flesh is smooth, the pathways of qì are free-flowing, and the movement of construction and defense never becomes abnormal. (2) For this reason, they are astute during the day and don't wake up at night. (3) In old people blood and qì are debilitated, the flesh is not smooth, and the pathways of construction and defense are inhibited. (4) For this reason, they are unable to be astute during the day and unable to sleep at night. (5) The fact that old people rest without sleeping and youngsters sleep without waking up is related to the superabundance and insufficiency of construction and defense and blood and qì."

II.9 The Forty-Seventh Difficulty
Sì shí qī nàn
四十七難

Line 1

人面獨能耐寒者，何也？

"Why is it that only the human face is able to withstand cold?"

Line 2

(一)然：人頭者諸陽之會也 。(二)諸陰脈皆至頸胸中而還 。(三)獨諸陽脈皆
上至頭耳 。(四)故令面耐寒也 。

(1) Answer: "A person's head is the meeting place of all yáng. (2) The various yīn vessels reach [only] the neck and chest and then return [to the lower part of the body]. (3) Only the various yáng vessels rise up and reach the head. (4) For this reason, the face is able to withstand cold."

II.10 The Forty-Ninth Difficulty
Sì shí jiǔ nàn
四十九難

Line 1

有正經自病，有五邪所傷，何以別之？

"There are illnesses that arise directly in the channels on their own, and there are [illnesses] that are caused by damage from the five evils. How do you distinguish between these?"

Line 2

(一)然：憂愁思慮則傷心；形寒飲冷則傷肺；恚怒氣逆，上而不下，則傷肝；飲食勞倦則傷脾；久坐濕地，強力入水，則傷腎。(二)是正經之自病也。

(1) Answer: "Anxiety, worry, thought, and preoccupation result in damage to the heart. A cold body and cool drinks result in damage to the lung. Rage and anger, causing the qì to move counterflow and ascend but not descend, result in damage to the liver. [Inappropriate] food and drink and taxation fatigue result in damage to the spleen. Prolonged sitting on damp ground and entering water after exertion result in damage to the kidney. (2) These are illnesses that arise directly in the channels on their own."

Line 3

何謂五邪？

"What are the so-called five evils?"

Line 4

(一)然：有中風，有傷暑，有飲食，有勞倦，有傷寒，有中濕，此之謂五邪 。(二)謝氏曰：飲食勞倦，自是二事 。(三)飲食得者，饑飽失時，此外邪傷也 。(四)勞倦得者，勞形力而致倦怠，此正經自病也 。

(1) Answer: "There is being struck by wind, damage from summer-heat, [inappropriate] food and drink, taxation fatigue, cold damage, and being struck by dampness. These are the so-called five evils. (2) Xiè said: '[Inappropriate] food and drink and taxation fatigue, these are two separate things. (3) The way you contract [illness due to inappropriate] food and drink is by starving or overeating in an untimely manner. This is [a case of] damage from external evil. (4) The way you contract taxation fatigue is by taxing your physical strength and thereby causing fatigue. This is [a case of] illness arising directly in the channel on its own.'"

Line 5

假令心病，何以知中風得之？

"Let us take illness in the heart as an example. How do we know when [illness in the heart] was contracted as a result of wind strike?"

Line 6

然：其色常赤 。何以言之？

Answer: "The patient's complexion will be red. Why do I say that?"

Line 7

(一)肝主色，自入為青，入心為赤，入脾為黃，入肺為白，入腎為黑 。(二)故知肝邪入心常赤色 。(三)其病身熱脅下滿痛，其脈浮大而弦 。

(1) The liver governs the complexion. When [evil] enters [the liver] itself, it manifests in a green-blue complexion. When it enters the heart, it manifests in a red complexion. When it enters the spleen, it manifests in a yellow complexion. When it enters the lung, it manifests in a white complexion. When it enters the kidney, it

manifests in a black complexion. (2) Therefore we know that when evil from the liver has entered the heart, it is normal to have a red complexion. (3) This illness manifests with generalized heat [effusion], fullness and pain below the rib-sides, and a floating, large, and stringlike pulse."

Line 8

何以知傷暑得之？

"How do I know when [a patient] has contracted [illness in the heart as the result of] summer-heat damage?"

Line 9

然：當惡臭。何以言之？

Answer: "The patient will exude a foul stench. Why do I say that?

Line 10

(一)心主臭，自入為焦臭，入脾為香臭，入肝為臊臭，入腎為腐臭。(二)故知心病當惡臭。(三)其病身熱而煩心痛，其脈浮大而散。

(1) The heart governs smells. When [evil] enters [the heart] itself, it manifests in a scorched smell. When it enters the spleen, it manifests in a fragrant smell. When it enters the liver, it manifests in a urine-like smell. When it enters the kidney, it manifests in a putrid smell. (2) Therefore we know that illness in the heart should [manifest] in a foul stench. (3) This illness manifests with generalized heat and heart vexation and pain, and a pulse that is floating, large, and a scattered pulse."

Line 11

何以知飲食勞倦得之？

"How do I know when [a patient] has contracted [illness in the heart as the result of inappropriate] food and drink and taxation fatigue?"

Line 12

然：當喜苦味也 。

Answer: "The patient will have a liking for bitter flavors.

Line 13

虛為不欲食，實為欲食 。何以言之？

Vacuity manifests in a lack of appetite. Repletion manifests in having an appetite. Why do I say that?

Line 14

(一)脾主味，入肝為酸，入心為苦，入肺為辛，入腎為鹹，自入為甘 。(二)故知脾邪入心，為喜苦味也 。(三)其病身熱而體重，嗜臥，四肢不收，其脈浮大而緩 。

(1) The spleen governs the flavors. When [evil] enters the liver, it manifests in sourness. When it enters the heart, it manifests in bitterness. When it enters the lung, it manifests in acridity. When it enters the kidney, it manifests in saltiness. When it enters [the spleen] itself, it manifests in sweetness. (2) Therefore we know that when evil from the spleen has entered the heart, it manifests in a liking for bitter flavors. (3) This illness manifests with generalized heat and a heavy body, somnolence, loss of use of the limbs, and a floating, large, and moderate pulse."

Line 15

何以知傷寒得之？

"How do I know when [a patient] has contracted [illness in the heart as the result of] cold damage?"

Line 16

然：當譫言妄語 。何以言之？

Answer: "The patient will have delirious raving. Why do I say that?

Line 17

(一)肺主聲，入肝為呼，入心為言，入脾為歌，入腎為呻，自入為哭 。(二)故知肺邪入心，為譫言妄語也 。(三)其病身熱，洒洒惡寒，甚則喘欬，其脈浮大而濇 。

(1) The lung governs sounds. When [evil] enters the liver, it manifests in shouting. When it enters the heart, it manifests in speaking. When it enters the spleen, it manifests in singing. When it enters the kidney, it manifests in groaning. When it enters [the lung] itself, it manifests in crying. (2) Therefore we know that when evil from the lung has entered the heart, it manifests in delirious raving. (3) This illness manifests with generalized heat, shivering with aversion to cold, in severe cases panting and cough, and a floating, large, and rough pulse."

Line 18

何以知中濕得之？

"How do I know when [a patient] has contracted [illness in the heart as the result of] being struck by dampness?"

Line 19

然：當喜汗出不可止 。何以言之？

Answer: "The patient will have a tendency to sweat incessantly. Why do I say that?

Line 20

(一)腎主液，入肝為泣，入心為汗，入脾為涎，入肺為涕，自入為唾 。(二) 故知腎邪入心，為汗出不可止也 。(三)其病身熱而少腹痛，足脛寒而逆，其 脈沉濡而大 。

(1) The kidney governs fluids. When [evil] enters the liver, it manifests in tears. When it enters the heart, it manifests in sweat. When it enters the spleen, it manifests in drool. When it enters the lung, it manifests in snivel. When it enters [the kidney] itself, it manifests in saliva. (2) Therefore we know that when evil from the kidney has entered the heart, it manifests in incessant sweating. (3) This illness manifests in generalized sweating and lesser abdominal pain, cold and counterflow in the feet and shins, and a sunken, soggy, and large pulse.

Line 21

此五邪之法也 。

These are the patterns of the five evils.

Line 22

(一)此篇越人蓋言陰陽 、臟腑 、經絡之偏虛偏實者也 。(二)由偏實也，故內 邪得而生；由偏虛也，故外邪得而入 。

(1) In this chapter, the person from Yuè discusses abnormal vacuity or repletion in yīn or yáng, in the viscera and bowels, and in the channels and network vessels. (2) As the result of abnormal repletion, illness is formed by contracting internal evil. As the results of abnormal vacuity, external evil is contracted and enters."

II.11 The Fiftieth Difficulty
Wǔ shí nàn
五十難

Line 1

病有虛邪，有實邪，有微邪，有賊邪，有正邪 。何以別之？

"Illness can be caused by vacuity evil, repletion evil, mild evil, bandit evil, and direct evil. How do we distinguish between these?"

Line 2

然：從後來者為虛邪；從前來者實邪；從所不勝來者為微邪；從所勝來者為賊邪；自病者為正邪 。

Answer: "If [the illness] comes from behind, it is a vacuity evil. If it comes from in front, it is a repletion evil. If it comes from not being overcome, it is a mild evil. If it comes from being overcome, it is a bandit evil. If the illness comes from itself, it is a direct evil.*

Note:

* I have chosen to simply translate this line literally. For a variety of explanations, see Unschuld, Nan-Ching, "The Fiftieth Difficult Issue," pp. 474-479. In the explanation proposed by Yáng Jìzhōu and demonstrated in the example of heart illness below, this line should be read as referring to the order of evils, as associated with the five viscera and phases in the theory of systematic correspondences. Hence, "comes from behind" refers to the organ/phase/type of evil that follows after the one associated with the present illness in the cycle of generation (shēng 生); "comes from in front" refers to the organ/phase/type of evil that precedes the one associated with the present illness. Similarly, "comes from not being overcome" and "comes from being overcome" refers to the order in the cycle of conquest (kè 克).

Line 3

(一)五行之道，生我者體。(二)其氣虛也，居吾之後而來為邪，故曰虛邪。(三)我生者相。(四)氣方實也，居吾之前而來為邪，故曰實邪。(五)正邪則本經自病者也。

(1) In the path of the five phases, what engenders me is the body. (2) If its qì is vacuous and what resides behind me comes as the evil, it is therefore called vacuity evil. (3) What I engender is the image. (4) If its qì is replete, and what resides in front of me comes as the evil, it is therefore called repletion evil. (5) A direct evil is then an illness that originates directly in the channel itself.

Line 4

何以言之？假令心病，中風得之為虛邪；傷暑得之為正邪；飲食勞倦得之為實邪；傷寒得之為微邪；中濕得之賊邪。

Why do I say this? Let us take illness in the heart as an example. If it is contracted as the result of wind strike, it is a repletion evil. If it is contracted as the result of summer-heat damage, it is a direct evil. If it is contracted as the result of food and drink and taxation fatigue, it is a repletion evil. If it is contracted as the result of cold damage, it is a minute evil. If it is contracted as the result of dampness strike, it is a bandit evil."

五邪舉心為例圖

Chart to show how the five evils act on the heart as an example

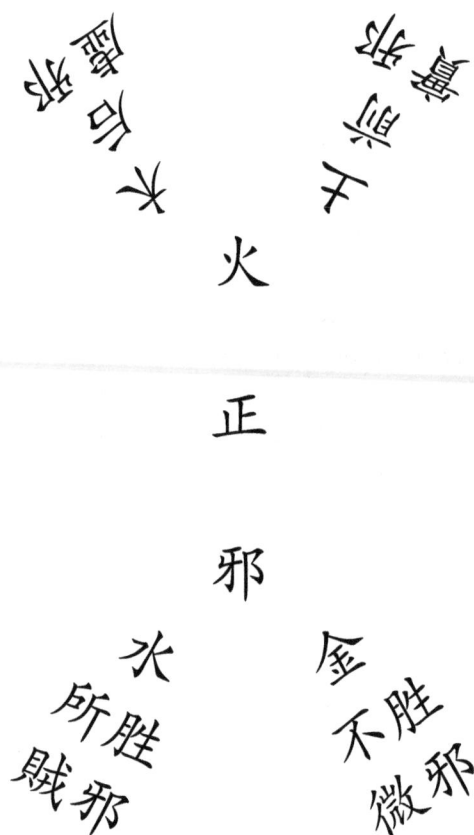

木不勝虛邪　　　土實邪

火

正

邪

水所勝賊邪　　金不勝微邪

II.12 The Fifty-First Difficulty
Wǔ shí yī nàn
五十一難

Line 1

病有欲得溫者，有欲得寒者；有欲得見人者，有不欲得見人者；而各不同，病在何臟腑也 。

"Among illnesses, there are those where [the patient] has a desire for warmth and those where [the patient] has a desire for cold; there are those where [the patient] has a desire to see people and those where [the patient] has an aversion to seeing people. Considering the difference in each of these [desires], which viscus or bowel is the illness located in?"

Line 2

然：病欲得寒欲見人者，病在腑也 。病欲得溫而不欲見人者，病在臟也 。

Answer: "When a condition is characterized by a desire for cold and for seeing people, the disease is located in the bowels. When a condition is characterized by a desire for warmth and an aversion to seeing people, the disease is located in the viscera.

Line 3

（一）何以言之？腑者陽也 。（二）陽病欲得寒，又欲見人 。（三）臟者陰也 。（四）陰病欲得溫，又欲閉戶獨處，惡聞人聲 。（五）故以別知臟腑之病也 。

(1) Why do I say this? The bowels are [associated with] yáng. (2) Yáng diseases are marked by a desire for cold and for seeing people. (3) The viscera are [associated with] yīn. (4) Yīn diseases are marked by a desire for warmth and for closing the doors and being left alone, and an aversion to hearing other people's sounds. (5) Therefore, we can use [these desires] to differentiate between diseases of the viscera and diseases of the bowels."

II.13 The Fifty-Second Difficulty
Wǔ shí èr nàn
五十二難

Line 1

腑臟發病，根本等否？

"As diseases develop in the viscera or bowels, are they essentially identical or not?"

Line 2

然：不等也

Answer: "They are not identical."

Line 3

何？

"How so?"

Line 4

(一)然：臟病者，正而不移 。其病不離其處 。(二)腑病者，彷彿賁嚮，上下行流，居處無常 。(三)故以此知臟腑根本不同也 。

(1) Answer: "Diseases of the viscera stay directly [in the affected viscus] and do not shift. These diseases do not leave their location. (2) Diseases in the bowels move back and forth, scurrying in all directions and flowing up and down. Their location is not permanent. (3) Therefore, we can use this [characteristic] to know that [diseases in] the viscera and bowels are essentially not identical."

II.14 The Fifty-Fifth Difficulty
Wǔ shí wǔ nàn
五十五難

Line 1

病有積有聚，何以別之？

"There is the disease of accumulations and the disease of gatherings. How do you distinguish between them?"

Line 2

然：積者陰氣也。聚者陽氣也。

Answer: "Accumulations are yīn qì. Gatherings are yáng qì.

Line 3

(一)故陰沉而伏，陽浮而動。(二)氣之所積名曰積，氣之所聚名曰聚。(三)故積者，五臟所生；聚者，六腑所成也。(四)積者陰氣也。其始發有常處，其痛不離其部，上下有所終始，左右有所窮處。(五)聚者陽氣也。其始發無根本，上下無所留止，其痛無常處，謂之聚。(六)故以是別知積聚也。

(1) Therefore yīn is sunken and hidden, yáng is floating and stirring. (2) Places where qì accumulates are called accumulations; places where qì gathers are called gatherings. (3) Therefore, accumulations are engendered by the five viscera; gatherings are formed by the six bowels. (4) Accumulations are yīn qì. They have a permanent location where they originally developed, their pain does not leave the section [of the body that the accumulation is located in], above and below they have a [distinct] beginning and end, and to the left and right they have places where they end. (5) Gatherings are yáng qì. They do not have roots in the location where they originally developed, above and below they do not have places where they stop and

stay, and their pain does not have a permanent location. These are referred to as gatherings. (6) Therefore, [you can] use [this characteristic] to distinguish between accumulations and gatherings.

II.15 The Fifty-Sixth Difficulty
Wǔ shí liù nàn
五十六難

Line 1

五臟之積，各有名乎？以何月何日得之？

"As for the accumulations of the five viscera, do they each have a name? Which month and which day are they contracted in?"

Line 2

(一)然：肝之積，名曰肥氣 。(二)在左脅下，如覆杯，有頭足，久不愈 。(三)令人發欬逆痎瘧，連歲不已 。(四)以季夏戊己日得之 。(五)何以言之？

(1) Answer: "Accumulations of the liver are called 'fat qì'. (2) They are located below the left rib-side, resemble an overturned cup, have a head and foot, and last a long time without improving. (3) They cause the person to suffer from cough and counterflow and malaria, and they do not cease year after year. (4) They are contracted in the last month of summer on an *wù jǐ* day. (5) Why do I say that?

Line 3

(一)肺病傳於肝，肝當傳脾 。(二)脾季夏適旺，旺不受邪 。(三)肝復欲還肺，肺不肯受，故留結為積 。(四)故知肥氣以季夏戊己日得之 。

(1) Lung disease is transmitted to the liver, and the liver should then transmit it to the spleen. (2) The spleen reaches its effulgence in the last month of summer. Being effulgent, it does not receive evils [during this time]. (3) The liver then turns around

and wants to return [the evil] to the lung, but the lung is unwilling to receive it. Therefore [the evil] remains [in the liver], binds, and forms an accumulation. (4) Therefore we know that 'fat qì' is contracted on an *wù jǐ* day in the last month of summer.

Line 4

（一）心之積曰伏梁 。（二）起臍上，大如臂，上至心下，久不愈 。（三）令人病煩心 。（四）以秋庚辛日得之 。（五）何以言之？

(1) Accumulations of the heart are called 'deep-lying beam'. (2) They start above the navel, are the size of an arm, rise up to below the heart, and last a long time without improving. (3) They cause the person to suffer from vexation in the heart. (4) They are contracted in autumn on a *gēng xīn* day. (5) Why do I say that?

Line 5

（一）腎病傳心，心當傳肺 。（二）肺以秋適旺，旺不受邪 。（三）心欲復還腎，腎不肯受，故留結為積 。（四）故知伏梁以秋庚辛日得之 。

(1) Kidney disease is transmitted to the heart, and the heart should then transmit it to the lung. (2) The lung reaches its effulgence in the autumn. Being effulgent, it does not receive evils [during this time]. (3) The heart then wants to turn around and return [the evil] to the kidney, but the kidney is unwilling to receive it. Therefore [the evil] remains [in the heart], binds, and forms an accumulation. (4) Therefore we know that 'deep-lying beam' is contracted on a *gēng xīn* day in autumn.

Line 6

（一）脾之積名曰痞氣 。（二）在胃脘，復大如盤，久不愈 。（三）令人四肢不收，發黃疸，飲食不為肌膚 。（四）以冬壬癸日得之 。（五）何以言之？

(1) Accumulations of the spleen are called 'glomus qì'. (2) They are located in the stomach duct, are several times the size of a plate, and last a long time without improving. (3) They cause the person to suffer from loss of use in the four limbs, development of jaundice, and failure to turn food and drink into muscle. (4) They are contracted in winter on a *rén guǐ* day. (5) Why do I say that?

Line 7

(一)肝病傳脾，脾當傳腎 。(二)腎以冬適旺，旺不受邪 。(三)脾復欲還肝，肝不肯受，故留結為積 。(四)故知痞氣以冬壬癸日得之 。

(1) Liver disease is transmitted to the spleen, and the spleen should then transmit it to the kidney. (2) The kidney reaches its effulgence in the winter. Being effulgent, it does not receive evils [during this time]. (3) The spleen then turns around and wants to return [the evil] to the liver, but the liver is unwilling to receive it. Therefore [the evil] remains [in the spleen], binds, and forms an accumulation. (4) Therefore we know that 'glomus qì' is contracted on a *rén guǐ* day in winter.

Line 8

(一)肺之積名曰息賁 。(二)在右脅下，復大如杯，久不已 。(三)令人洒淅寒熱，喘欬，發肺癰 。(四)以春甲乙日得之 。(五)何以言之？

(1) Accumulations of the lung are called 'stopping and running.'* (2) They are located below the right rib-side, are several times the size of a cup, and last a long time without stopping. (3) They cause the person to suffer from shivering with [aversion to] cold and heat [effusion], panting and cough, and the development of pulmonary welling-abscesses. (4) They are contracted in the spring on a *jiǎ yǐ* day. (5) Why do I say that?

Note:

> * Reading *xī* 息 as "respiration," Wiseman and Feng translate this term as "rushing respiration," based on the symptoms associated with this type of accumulation, namely "hasty rapid breathing with qì rushing counterflow upward" (*A Practical Dictionary*, 510). I have chosen to follow the mainstream commentary traditions of the present text as well as the *Nàn Jīng* instead, which interpret *xī* 息 here in a different sense as "to stop/rest," i.e. the opposite of *bēn* 賁. The term then has the meaning of an accumulation that sometimes is motionless and at other times is "running around."

Line 9

(一)心病傳肺，肺當得肝 。(二)肝以春適旺，旺不受邪 。(三)肺復欲還心，心不肯受，故留結為積 。(四)故知息賁以春甲乙日得之 。

(1) Heart disease is transmitted to the lung, and the lung should then transmit it to the liver. (2) The liver reaches its effulgence in the spring. Effulgent, it does not receive evils [during this time]. (3) The lung then turns around and wants to return [the evil] to the heart, but the heart is unwilling to receive it. Therefore [the evil] remains [in the lung], binds, and forms an accumulation. (4) Therefore we know that 'stopping and running' is contracted on a *jiǎ yǐ* day in the spring.

Line 10

(一)腎之積名曰賁豚 。(二)發於少腹，上至心下，若豚狀，或上或下無時，久不已 。(三)令人喘逆，骨痿少氣 。(四)以夏丙丁日得之 。(五)何以言之？

(1) Accumulations of the kidney are called 'running piglet'. (2) They develop in the lower abdomen, rise up to below the heart, resemble a piglet in they way that they run up and down unpredictably, and last a long time without stopping. (3) They cause the person to suffer from panting with counterflow, bone wilting, and shortage of qì. (4) They are contracted in summer on a *bǐng dīng* day. (5) Why do I say that?

Line 11

(一)脾病傳腎，腎當傳心 。(二)以夏適旺，旺不受邪 。(三)腎復欲還脾，脾不肯受，故留為積 。(四)故知賁豚以夏丙丁日得之 。

(1) Spleen disease is transmitted to the kidney, and the kidney should then transmit it to the heart. (2) [The heart] reaches its effulgence in the summer. Effulgent, it does not receive evils [during this time]. (3) The kidney then turns around and wants to return [the evil] to the spleen, but the spleen is unwilling to receive it. Therefore [the evil] remains [in the kidney] and forms an accumulation. (4) Therefore we know that 'running piglet' is contracted on a *bǐng dīng* day in summer.

Line 12

此五積之要法也 。

These are the major patterns of the five accumulations."

II.16 The Fifty-Ninth Difficulty
Wǔ shí jiǔ nàn
五十九難

Line 1

狂癲之病，何以別之？

"How do you distinguish between mania and withdrawal?"

Line 2

(一)然：狂疾之始發，少臥而不饑，自高賢也，自辨智也，自倨貴也，妄笑好歌樂，妄行不休是也 。(二)癲疾始發，意不樂，僵仆直視，其脈三部陰陽俱盛是也 。

(1) Answer: "The initial development of mania disease manifests with reduced sleep and lack of hunger; with overestimating oneself as a person of great virtue, great wisdom, and great value; with laughing wildly and a liking for singing and music; and with running wildly without resting. (2) The initial development of withdrawal manifests with a joyless state of mind, with sudden collapse and rigid staring, and with a pulse that is exuberant in all three yīn and yáng sections."

II.17 The Sixtieth Difficulty
Liù shí nàn
六十難

Line 1

頭心之病，有厥痛，有真痛，何謂也？

"Among diseases of the head and heart, we speak of 'reversal pain' and of 'true pain'. What does this refer to?"

Line 2

(一)然：手三陽之脈受風寒，伏留而不去者，則名厥頭痛 。(二)入連在腦者，名真頭痛 。(三)其五臟氣相干，名厥心痛 。(四)其痛甚，但在心，手足青者，即名真心痛 。(五)其真頭、心痛者，旦發夕死，夕發旦死 。

(1) Answer: "When the three yáng vessels of the hand contract wind-cold, and [this evil] becomes deep-lying and lodged instead of leaving, we call this 'reversal headache'. (2) When it enters and connects with the brain, we call it 'true headache'. (3) When a person's [evil] qì in the five viscera interferes [with the heart, causing pain there], we call it 'reversal heart pain'. (4) When the pain is severe but limited only to the heart and it is accompanied by green-blue hands and feet, we call it 'true heart pain'. (5) When true head or heart pain develop at dawn, the patient will die at dusk; when it develops at dusk, the patient will die at dawn."

II.18 The Sixty-First Difficulty
Liù shí yī nàn

六十一難

Line 1

經言望而知之謂之神；聞而知之謂之聖；問而知之謂之工；切脈而知之謂之巧。何謂也？

"When the classic says 'to know by looking is divine, to know by listening is sagely, to know by asking is crafty, to know by taking the pulse is skillful,' what does this mean?"

Line 2

(一)然：望而知之者，望見其五色，以知其病。(二)素問五臟生成篇云：色見青如草滋，黃如枳實，黑如炲，赤如衃血，白如枯骨者，皆死。(三)青如翠羽，赤如雞冠，黃如蟹腹，白如豕膏，黑如烏翎者，皆生。(四)靈樞云：青黑為痛，黃赤為熱，白為寒。(五)又云：赤色出於兩顴，大如拇指者，病雖小愈，必卒死。(六)黑色出於庭，大如拇指，必不病而卒。(七)又云：診血脈者多赤，多熱；多青，多痛；多黑為久痹。(八)多黑多赤多青皆見者，為寒熱，身痛。(九)面色微黃，齒垢黃，爪甲上黃，黃疸也。(十)又如驗產婦，面赤舌青，母活子死；面青舌赤，沫出，母死子活；唇口俱青，子母俱死之類也。

(1) Answer: "'To know by looking' means to know a patient's disease from seeing the five colors.[1] (2) A quotation from the *Sù Wèn* chapter 'On the Engenderment of the Five Viscera'[2] states: 'Whenever you see a complexion that is green-blue like grass sprouting, yellow like dried unripe bitter orange, black like smoky soot, red like coagulated blood, or white like desiccated bones, it always means death. (3) [Whenever you see a complexion that is] green-blue like the feathers of the kingfisher, red like a rooster's comb, yellow like a crab's abdomen, white like pork lard, or black like crow's feathers, it always means life.' (4) A quotation from the *Líng Shū* states: 'A green-blue or black [complexion] means pain, a yellow or red [complexion] means

heat, a white [complexion] means cold.' (5) Another quotation: 'If you see redness emanating from both cheeks, in an area the size of a thumb, even though the illness will show minor improvement, the patient will invariably die all of a sudden. (6) If you see blackness emanating from the face, in an area the size of a thumb, the patient will invariably not be sick and yet die all of a sudden.' (7) Another quotation: 'When examining the blood vessels, increased redness means increased heat. Increased green-blue coloration means increased pain. Increased blackness means chronic impediment. (8) Increased black, red, and green-blue coloration all at the same time means [aversion to] cold, heat [effusion], and generalized pain. (9) If the complexion in the face is slightly yellow, if there are yellow deposits on the teeth, and if there is yellowness on the nails of the fingers and toes, this is jaundice.' (10) Another: 'When examining a woman going into labor, if the face is red and the tongue green-blue, the mother will live but the child die. If the face is green-blue, the tongue red, and she is foaming at the mouth, the mother will die but the child live. If the lips and mouth are both green-blue, the child and mother will both die.'

Notes:

1. I.e. to diagnose a patient's illness on the basis of the perceived skin complexion.
2. *Sù Wèn* 10.

Line 3

(一)聞而知之者，聞其五音，以別其病 。(二)四明陳氏曰：五臟有聲，而聲有音 。(三)肝聲呼，音應角，調而直，音聲相應則無病；角亂則病在肝 。(四)心聲笑，音應徵，和而長，音聲相應則無病；微亂則病在心 。(五)脾聲歌，音應宮，大而和，音聲相應則無病；宮亂則病在脾 。(六)肺聲哭，音應商，輕而勁，音聲相應則無病；商亂則病在肺 。(七)腎聲呻，音應羽，沈而深，音聲相應則無病；羽亂則病在腎 。

(1) 'To know by listening' means to differentiate the patient's disease by listening to the five sounds. (2) Chén Sì-míng says: 'The five viscera have sounds [associated with them], and the sounds have musical notes [associated with them]. (3) The liver's sound is shouting, and the corresponding note is *jué*, which should be balanced and straight. When the note and sound correspond to each other, there is no disease. When *jué* is disordered, the disease is in the liver. (4) The heart's sound is laughter, and the corresponding note is *zhǐ*, which should be harmonious and long. When the note and sound correspond to each other, there is no disease. When *zhǐ* is disordered, the disease is in the heart. (5) The spleen's sound is singing, and the cor-

responding note is *gōng*, which should be large and harmonious. When the note and sound correspond to each other, there is no disease. When *gōng* is disordered, the disease is in the spleen. (6) The lung's sound is crying, and the corresponding note is *shāng*, which should be light and vigorous. When the note and sound correspond to each other, there is no disease. When *shāng* is disordered, the disease is in the lung. (7) The kidney's sound is groaning, and the corresponding note is *yǔ*, which should be sunken and deep. When the note and sound correspond to each other, there is no disease. When *yǔ* is disordered, the disease is in the kidney.'

Line 4

(一)問而知之者，問其所欲五味，以知其病所起所在也 。(二)靈樞云：五味入口，各有所走，各有所病 。(三)酸走筋，多食之令人癃 。(四)鹹走血，多食之令人渴 。(五)辛走氣，多食之令人洞心 。(六)辛與氣俱行，故辛入心而與汗俱出 。(七)苦走骨，多食之令人變嘔 。(八)甘走肉，多食之令人悗心 。(九)推此則知 。(十)問其所欲五味，以知其病之所起，所在也 。(十一)袁氏曰：問其所欲五味中偏嗜偏多食之物，則知臟氣有偏勝偏絕之候也 。

(1) 'To know by asking' means to know the origin and present location of a disease by asking the patient which of the five flavors he or she desires. (2) A quotation from the *Líng Shū* states: 'As the five flavors enter the mouth, each has a specific location where it goes to and a specific disease [associated with it]. (3) Sourness goes into the sinews and, when consumed in excess, causes the person to suffer from dribbling urinary block. (4) Saltiness goes into the blood and, when consumed in excess, causes the person to suffer from thirst. (5) Acridity goes into the qì and, when consumed in excess, causes the person to suffer from a hollowed-out feeling in the heart. (6) Acridity and qì flow together. Therefore acridity enters the heart and exits together with sweat. (7) Bitterness goes into the bones and, when consumed in excess, causes the person to suffer from vomiting. (8) Sweetness goes into the flesh and, when consumed in excess, causes the person to suffer from oppression in the heart.' (9) By deducing these [connections], [the physician can] know [the disease]. (10) By asking the patient which of the five flavors he or she desires, we can know where the disease originated and where it is located. (11) Yuán said: 'By inquiring after the patient's abnormal cravings and foods that he or she has consumed in abnormal excesses among the five flavors the patient desires, we know the symptoms [to recognize] which of the five visceral qì is abnormally prevalent or expired.'

Line 5

(一)切脈而知之者，診其寸口，視其虛實，以知其病，病在何臟腑也。(二)診寸口，即第一難之義。(三)王氏之脈法讚曰：脈有三部，尺、寸及關，榮衛流行，不失衡銓。(四)腎沉、心洪、肺浮、肝弦，此自常經，不失銖錢。(五)出入升降，漏刻周旋。(六)水下二刻，脈一周身，旋復寸口，虛實見焉。(七)經言以外知之曰聖，以內知之曰神，此之謂也。(八)以外知之，望聞；以內知之，問切也。

(1) 'To know by taking the pulse' means to know the patient's disease and to know which viscus or bowel the disease is located in by examining [the pulse at] the *cùn kǒu* and observing its state of vacuity or repletion. (2) Examining at the *cùn kǒu* is explained in the First Difficulty.* (3) A quote from Wáng's 'In Praise of the Pulse Method': 'The pulse has three sections, the *chǐ*, *cùn*, and *guān*. The flow of construction and defense [qì] does not depart from [the accuracy of] a steelyard balance. (4) The kidney [pulse] is sunken, the heart [pulse] is surging, the lung [pulse] is floating, the liver [pulse] is stringlike. These are the pulses coming from the standard channels, which do not depart even by the tiniest weight. (5) Entering and exiting, ascending and descending, [like water] dripping in the markings [of the water clock], they revolve in their cycle. (6) As the water drips down two markings [in the water clock], the pulse completes one cycle through the body and returns back to the *cùn kǒu*. Hence vacuity and repletion can be discerned in it.' (7) This is the meaning of the statement from the classic that 'to know [illness] from external [signs] is sagely, but to know it from internal [signs] is divine'. (8) To know [illness] from external [signs] refers to looking and listening. To know [illness] from internal [signs] refers to asking and taking the pulse.

Note:

* A reference to the first chapter of the *Nàn Jīng*, translated and explained in Unschuld, *Nan-Ching. The Classic of Difficult Issues*, pp. 65-90. See also above, chapter II.1 on the First Difficult Issue, pp. 170-173.

Line 6

(一)神，微妙也。(二)聖，通明也。

(1) Divine means wondrously subtle. (2) Sagely means penetrating and perceptive.

Book Index

wǔ shí jiǔ cì	五十九刺	the 59 needles	45
wǔ yùn liù qì	五運六氣	five movements and six qì	144
wù hán	惡寒	aversion to cold	82
xī	息	to stop/rest	200
xià	下	below the diaphragm/ lower half of the body	93
xiǎo xīn	小心	lit. "small heart"	133
xīn zhī gài yě	心之蓋也	canopy of the heart	40
xíng	形	physical body	92
xǔ	呴	to breathe on	179
xuè	血	blood	92
yāo	夭	to perish	34
yāo fǎn zhé	腰反折	arched-back lumbus	57
yín shí	寅時	the time between 3 and 5 a.m., i.e. daybreak.	123
yōng	癰	welling-abscess	
yù	愈	heal	79
zǎo shí	早食	breakfast	142
zàng	臟	viscus	74, 88
zàng huì	臟會	meeting point of the viscera	74
zhēn	針	needle	29, 55
zhì	志	will	92
zhì wèi bìng	治未病	treat disease before it arises	169

針灸大成・卷之一

Alternate point names are in ( )'s

Points Index

213

Indications Index

針灸大成・卷之一

Indications Index

針灸大成・卷之一

General Index

220

針灸大成 · 卷之一

The Chinese Medicine Database

www.cm-db.com

The Chinese Medicine Database has been organized around one central principle -- translation of Classical Chinese texts, and dissemination of that information.

There are thousands of Chinese medicine texts that have never been translated. We have compiled a small list on our website of the ones that we have found, but we believe that there are tens of thousands of documents that span from pre-Republican times to the Han dynasty. Most of these documents will never be read by people in the West, simply because of lack of translation.

We have created a vehicle, that allows interested practitioners, students, institutions, and scholars to help support and fund the translation of these documents, and then mine and synthesize the data that is gained from these texts.

The Database contains:

Monographs on:
669 Single Herbs
1485 Formulas
Mayway's Patents
ITM's Formulations
Golden Flowers Formulations
Health Concerns Formulations
Blue Poppy's Patents
Classical Pearls Formulations by Heiner Fruehauf
OBGYN Modifications to Formulas
Single Points: the 361 Regular Points

15,000 Western Diagnoses with ICD-9 Codes

A Chinese-English dictionary:
Containing over 100,000 terms, including the Eastland and the WHO term sets.

A Western Book search containing:
Fenners Complete Formulary
    by B. Fenner
The 1918 Dispensatory of the United States of America
    Edited by Joseph P. Remington, Horatio C. Woods and others
The Eclectic Materia Medica, Pharmacology and Therapeutics
    by Harvey Wickes Felter, M.D.

A Personal Dashboard, which allows users to:
Blog
Take notes on any monograph.
Search for other users by city, state, country and name.
Make friends all around the world.

Share and compare notes with friends.

Personalize your dashboard by adding photos, and information about your practice.

Translations:

Shāng Hán Lái Sū Jí 傷寒來蘇集: Renewal of Treatise on Cold Damage

Qí Jīng Bā Mài Kǎo 奇經八脈考: Explanation of the Eight Vessels of the Marvellous Meridians

Shāng Hán Míng Lǐ Lùn 傷寒明理論: Treatise on Enlightening the Principles of Cold Damage.

Wú Jū Tōng Yī àn 吴鞠通医案: Case Studies of Wú Jū-tōng

The Nán Jīng 難經: The Classic of Difficulties

The Zang Fu Biao Ben Han Re Xu Shi Yong Yao Shi 臟腑標本寒熱虛實用藥式: Viscera and Bowels, Tip and Root, Cold and Heat, Vacuity and Repletion Model for Using Medicinals

Bèi Jí Qiān Jīn Yào Fāng 備急千金要方: Essential Prescriptions Worth a Thousand Gold Pieces For Emergencies. vol. 2-4

Wēn Rè Lún 溫熱論: Treatise on Warm Heat Disease

Shāng Hán Shé Jiàn 傷寒舌鑒: Tongue Mirror of Cold Damage

Xǔ Shì Yī àn 許氏醫案: Case Histories of Master Xu

Fǔ Xìng Jué Zāng Fǔ Yòng Yào Fǎ Yào 輔行決臟腑用藥法要: Secret Instructions for Assisting the Body: Essential Methods for the Application of Drugs to the Viscera & Bowels

Biāo Yōu Fù (annotation) 標幽賦（楊氏註解）: Indicating the Obscure

Liú Juān Zǐ Guǐ Yí Fāng 劉涓子鬼遺方: Liu Juanzi's Formulas Inherited from Ghosts

Shèn Jí Chú Yán 慎疾芻言: Precautions in Illness: My Humble Thoughts

Yào Zhèng Jì Yí 藥症忌宜: Medicinals & Patterns Contraindications & Appropriate [Choices]

Benefits:

Subscribers to the Database receive a 10% discount on our published books when they are in pre-release.

Subscribers are eligible to win our annual drawing of $1,000.00 worth of debt repayment*.

(To be eligible subscribers must have subscribed prior to the month of November prior to the year of the drawing, and keep their billing current through the next 9 months. *Debt repayment means for credit card debt or student loan debt.)

We translate texts as often, and in quantities that reflect our user base. The larger amount of subscribers that we have, the more translation that we can accomplish. This project is only successful because of individuals like yourself who want to read more of the Classics of Chinese medicine.

Published Books:

2008 Bèi Jí Qiān Jīn Yào Fāng 備急千金要方: Essential Prescriptions Worth a Thousand Gold Pieces For Emergencies. vol. 2-4 by Sūn Sī Miǎo 孫思邈
Translated by Sabine Wilms.
ISBN 978-0-9799552-0-4

2010 Zhēn Jiǔ Dà Chéng 針灸大成: The Great Compendium of Acupuncture & Moxabustion vol. V by Yáng Jì Zhōu 楊繼州
Translated by Lorraine Wilcox.
ISBN 978-0-9799552-4-2

Forthcoming Zhēn Jiǔ Dà Chéng 針灸大成: The Great Compendium of Acupuncture & Moxabustion vol. 2-4 by Yáng Jì Zhōu 楊繼州
Translated by Shelley Ochs L.Ac.

9 780979 955228